Springer Series in S

MW00806703

Advisors:
P. Bickel, P. Diggle, S. Fienberg, K. Krickeberg,
I. Olkin, N. Wermuth, S. Zeger

Springer
New York
Berlin
Heidelberg
Barcelona
Hong Kong
London
Milan
Paris
Singapore
Tokyo

Springer Series in Statistics

Andersen/Borgan/Gill/Keiding: Statistical Models Based on Counting Processes.
Atkinson/Riani: Robust Diagnotstic Regression Analysis.
Berger: Statistical Decision Theory and Bayesian Analysis, 2nd edition.
Borg/Groenen: Modern Multidimensional Scaling: Theory and Applications
Brockwell/Davis: Time Series: Theory and Methods, 2nd edition.
Chan/Tong: Chaos: A Statistical Perspective.
Chen/Shao/Ibrahim: Monte Carlo Methods in Bayesian Computation.
David/Edwards: Annotated Readings in the History of Statistics.
Devroye/Lugosi: Combinatorial Methods in Density Estimation.
Efromovich: Nonparametric Curve Estimation: Methods, Theory, and Applications.
Eggermont/LaRiccia: Maximum Penalized Likelihood Estimation, Volume I:
    Density Estimation.
Fahrmeir/Tutz: Multivariate Statistical Modelling Based on Generalized Linear
    Models, 2nd edition.
Farebrother: Fitting Linear Relationships: A History of the Calculus of Observations
    1750-1900.
Federer: Statistical Design and Analysis for Intercropping Experiments, Volume I:
    Two Crops.
Federer: Statistical Design and Analysis for Intercropping Experiments, Volume II:
    Three or More Crops.
Fisher/Sen: The Collected Works of Wassily Hoeffding.
Glaz/Naus/Wallenstein: Scan Statistics.
Good: Permutation Tests: A Practical Guide to Resampling Methods for Testing
    Hypotheses, 2nd edition.
Gouriéroux: ARCH Models and Financial Applications.
Gu: Smoothing Spline ANOVA Models.
Haberman: Advanced Statistics, Volume I: Description of Populations.
Hall: The Bootstrap and Edgeworth Expansion.
Härdle: Smoothing Techniques: With Implementation in S.
Harrell: Regression Modeling Strategies: With Applications to Linear Models,
    Logistic Regression, and Survival Analysis
Hart: Nonparametric Smoothing and Lack-of-Fit Tests.
Hastie/Tibshirani/Friedman: The Elements of Statistical Learning: Data Mining,
    Inference, and Prediction
Hedayat/Sloane/Stufken: Orthogonal Arrays: Theory and Applications.
Heyde: Quasi-Likelihood and its Application: A General Approach to Optimal
    Parameter Estimation.
Huet/Bouvier/Gruet/Jolivet: Statistical Tools for Nonlinear Regression: A Practical
    Guide with S-PLUS Examples.
Ibrahim/Chen/Sinha: Bayesian Survival Analysis.
Kolen/Brennan: Test Equating: Methods and Practices.
Kotz/Johnson (Eds.): Breakthroughs in Statistics Volume I.
Kotz/Johnson (Eds.): Breakthroughs in Statistics Volume II.
Kotz/Johnson (Eds.): Breakthroughs in Statistics Volume III.

(continued after index)

J.O. Ramsay
B.W. Silverman

Applied Functional Data Analysis

Methods and Case Studies

With 112 Figures

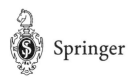 Springer

J.O. Ramsay
Department of Psychology
McGill University
Montreal, Quebec H3A 1B1
Canada
ramsay@psych.mcgill.ca

B.W. Silverman
Department of Mathematics
University of Bristol
Bristol BS8 1TW
United Kingdom
b.w.silverman@bristol.ac.uk

Library of Congress Cataloging-in-Publication Data
Ramsay, J.O. (James O).
    Applied functional data analysis : methods and case studies / J.O. Ramsay, B.W. Silverman.
      p. cm. — (Springer series in statistics)
    Includes bibliographical references and index.
    ISBN 0-387-95414-7 (pbk. : alk. paper)
      1. Multivariate analysis. I. Silverman, B.W., 1952– II. Title. III. Series.
QA278 .R35 2002
519.5'35—dc21   2002022924

ISBN 0-387-95414-7   Printed on acid-free paper.

Printed in the United States of America.

9 8 7 6 5 4 3 2 1   SPIN 10862137

Typesetting: Pages created by the authors using a Springer TEX macro package.

www.springer-ny.com

Springer-Verlag   New York Berlin Heidelberg
A member of BertelsmannSpringer Science+Business Media GmbH

Preface

Almost as soon as we had completed our previous book *Functional Data Analysis* in 1997, it became clear that potential interest in the field was far wider than the audience for the thematic presentation we had given there. At the same time, both of us rapidly became involved in relevant new research involving many colleagues in fields outside statistics.

This book treats the field in a different way, by considering case studies arising from our own collaborative research to illustrate how functional data analysis ideas work out in practice in a diverse range of subject areas. These include criminology, economics, archaeology, rheumatology, psychology, neurophysiology, auxology (the study of human growth), meteorology, biomechanics, and education—and also a study of a juggling statistician.

Obviously such an approach will not cover the field exhaustively, and in any case functional data analysis is not a hard-edged closed system of thought. Nevertheless we have tried to give a flavor of the range of methodology we ourselves have considered. We hope that our personal experience, including the fun we had working on these projects, will inspire others to extend "functional" thinking to many other statistical contexts. Of course, many of our case studies required development of existing methodology, and readers should gain the ability to adapt methods to their own problems too.

No previous knowledge of functional data analysis is needed to read this book, and although it complements our previous book in some ways, neither is a prerequisite for the other. We hope it will be of interest, and accessible, both to statisticians and to those working in other fields. Similarly, it should appeal both to established researchers and to students coming to the subject for the first time.

Functional data analysis is very much involved with computational statistics, but we have deliberately not written a computer manual or cookbook. Instead, there is an associated Web site accessible from `www.springer-ny.com` giving annotated analyses of many of the data sets, as well as some of the data themselves. The languages of these analyses are MATLAB, R, or S-PLUS, but the aim of the analyses is to explain the computational thinking rather than to provide a package, so they should be useful for those who use other languages too. We have, however, freely used a library of functions that we developed in these languages, and these may be downloaded from the Web site.

In both our books, we have deliberately set out to present a personal account of this rapidly developing field. Some specialists will, no doubt, notice omissions of the kind that are inevitable in this kind of presentation, or may disagree with us about the aspects to which we have given most emphasis. Nevertheless, we hope that they will find our treatment interesting and stimulating. One of our reasons for making the data, and the analyses, available on the Web site is our wish that others may do better. Indeed, may others write better books!

There are many people to whom we are deeply indebted. Particular acknowledgment is due to the distinguished paleopathologist Juliet Rogers, who died just before the completion of this book. Among much other research, Juliet's long-term collaboration with BWS gave rise to the studies in Chapters 4 and 8 on the shapes of the bones of arthritis sufferers of many centuries ago. Michael Newton not only helped intellectually, but also gave us some real data by allowing his juggling to be recorded for analysis in Chapter 12. Others whom we particularly wish to thank include Darrell Bock, Virginia Douglas, Zmira Elbaz-King, Theo Gasser, Vince Gracco, Paul Gribble, Michael Hermanussen, John Kimmel, Craig Leth-Steenson, Xiaochun Li, Nicole Malfait, David Ostry, Tim Ramsay, James Ramsey, Natasha Rossi, Lee Shepstone, Matthew Silverman, and Xiaohui Wang. Each of them made a contribution essential to some aspect of the work we report, and we apologize to others we have neglected to mention by name. We are very grateful to the Stanford Center for Advanced Study in the Behavioral Sciences, the American College Testing Program, and to the McGill students in the Psychology 747A seminar on functional data analysis. We also thank all those who provided comments on our software and pointed out problems.

Montreal, Quebec, Canada   Jim Ramsay
Bristol, United Kingdom   Bernard Silverman
January 2002

Contents

Preface   **v**

1 Introduction   **1**
   1.1   Why consider functional data at all?   1
   1.2   The Web site   2
   1.3   The case studies   2
   1.4   How is functional data analysis distinctive?   14
   1.5   Conclusion and bibliography   15

2 Life Course Data in Criminology   **17**
   2.1   Criminology life course studies   17
      2.1.1   Background   17
      2.1.2   The life course data   18
   2.2   First steps in a functional approach   19
      2.2.1   Turning discrete values into a functional datum .   19
      2.2.2   Estimating the mean   21
   2.3   Functional principal component analyses   23
      2.3.1   The basic methodology   23
      2.3.2   Smoothing the PCA   26
      2.3.3   Smoothed PCA of the criminology data   26
      2.3.4   Detailed examination of the scores   28
   2.4   What have we seen?   31

2.5   How are functions stored and processed?   33
    2.5.1   Basis expansions   33
    2.5.2   Fitting basis coefficients to the observed data . .   35
    2.5.3   Smoothing the sample mean function   36
    2.5.4   Calculations for smoothed functional PCA   37
2.6   Cross-validation for estimating the mean   38
2.7   Notes and bibliography   40

3   The Nondurable Goods Index   **41**
3.1   Introduction   41
3.2   Transformation and smoothing   43
3.3   Phase-plane plots   44
3.4   The nondurable goods cycles   47
3.5   What have we seen?   54
3.6   Smoothing data for phase-plane plots   55
    3.6.1   Fourth derivative roughness penalties   55
    3.6.2   Choosing the smoothing parameter   55

4   Bone Shapes from a Paleopathology Study   **57**
4.1   Archaeology and arthritis   57
4.2   Data capture   58
4.3   How are the shapes parameterized?   59
4.4   A functional principal components analysis   61
    4.4.1   Procrustes rotation and PCA calculation   61
    4.4.2   Visualizing the components of shape variability .   61
4.5   Varimax rotation of the principal components   63
4.6   Bone shapes and arthritis: Clinical relationship?   65
4.7   What have we seen?   66
4.8   Notes and bibliography   66

5   Modeling Reaction-Time Distributions   **69**
5.1   Introduction   69
5.2   Nonparametric modeling of density functions   71
5.3   Estimating density and individual differences   73
5.4   Exploring variation across subjects with PCA   76
5.5   What have we seen?   79
5.6   Technical details   80

6   Zooming in on Human Growth   **83**
6.1   Introduction   83
6.2   Height measurements at three scales   84
6.3   Velocity and acceleration   86
6.4   An equation for growth   89
6.5   Timing or phase variation in growth   91
6.6   Amplitude and phase variation in growth   93

6.7		What we have seen?	96
6.8		Notes and further issues	97
	6.8.1	Bibliography	97
	6.8.2	The growth data	98
	6.8.3	Estimating a smooth monotone curve to fit data .	98

7 Time Warping Handwriting and Weather Records   101

7.1	Introduction	101
7.2	Formulating the registration problem	102
7.3	Registering the printing data	104
7.4	Registering the weather data	105
7.5	What have we seen?	110
7.6	Notes and references	110
	7.6.1 Continuous registration	110
	7.6.2 Estimation of the warping function	113

8 How Do Bone Shapes Indicate Arthritis?   115

8.1	Introduction	115
8.2	Analyzing shapes without landmarks	116
8.3	Investigating shape variation	120
	8.3.1 Looking at means alone	120
	8.3.2 Principal components analysis	120
8.4	The shape of arthritic bones	123
	8.4.1 Linear discriminant analysis	123
	8.4.2 Regularizing the discriminant analysis	125
	8.4.3 Why not just look at the group means?	127
8.5	What have we seen?	128
8.6	Notes and further issues	128
	8.6.1 Bibliography	128
	8.6.2 Why is regularization necessary?	129
	8.6.3 Cross-validation in classification problems	130

9 Functional Models for Test Items   131

9.1	Introduction	131
9.2	The ability space curve	132
9.3	Estimating item response functions	135
9.4	PCA of log odds-ratio functions	136
9.5	Do women and men perform differently on this test?	138
9.6	A nonlatent trait: Arc length	140
9.7	What have we seen?	143
9.8	Notes and bibliography	143

10 Predicting Lip Acceleration from Electromyography   145

10.1	The neural control of speech	145
10.2	The lip and EMG curves	147

10.3   The linear model for the data 148
10.4   The estimated regression function 150
10.5   How far back should the historical model go? 152
10.6   What have we seen? 155
10.7   Notes and bibliography 155

11 The Dynamics of Handwriting Printed Characters   **157**
11.1   Recording handwriting in real time 157
11.2   An introduction to dynamic models 158
11.3   One subject's printing data 160
11.4   A differential equation for handwriting 162
11.5   Assessing the fit of the equation 165
11.6   Classifying writers by using their dynamic equations . . 166
11.7   What have we seen? 170

12 A Differential Equation for Juggling   **171**
12.1   Introduction 171
12.2   The data and preliminary analyses 172
12.3   Features in the average cycle 173
12.4   The linear differential equation 176
12.5   What have we seen? 180
12.6   Notes and references 181

References   **183**

Index   **187**

1
Introduction

1.1   Why consider functional data at all?

Functional data come in many forms, but their defining quality is that they consist of functions—often, but not always, smooth curves. In this book, we consider functional data arising in many different fields, ranging from the shapes of bones excavated by archaeologists, to economic data collected over many years, to the path traced out by a juggler's finger. The fundamental aims of the analysis of functional data are the same as those of more conventional statistics: to formulate the problem at hand in a way amenable to statistical thinking and analysis; to develop ways of presenting the data that highlight interesting and important features; to investigate variability as well as mean characteristics; to build models for the data observed, including those that allow for dependence of one observation or variable on another, and so on.

We have chosen case studies to cover a wide range of fields of application, and one of our aims is to demonstrate how large is the potential scope of functional data analysis. If you work through all the case studies you will have covered a broad sweep of existing methods in functional data analysis and, in some cases, you will study new methodology developed for the particular problem in hand. But more importantly, we hope that the readers will gain an insight into functional ways of thinking.

What sort of data come under the general umbrella of functional data? In some cases, the original observations are interpolated from longitudinal data, quantities observed as they evolve through time. However, there are many other ways that functional data can arise. For instance, in our study of children with attention deficit hyperactivity disorder, we take a large number of independent numerical observations for each child, and the functional datum for that child is the estimated probability density of these observations. Sometimes our data are curves traced out on a surface or in space. The juggler's finger directly traces out the data we analyze in that case, but in another example, on the characteristics of examination questions, the functional data arise as part of the modeling process. In the archaeological example, the shape of a two-dimensional image of each bone is the functional datum in question. And of course images as well as curves can appear as functional data or as functional parameters in models, as we show in our study of electromyography recordings and speech articulation.

The field of functional data analysis is still in its infancy, and the boundaries between functional data analysis and other aspects of statistics are definitely fuzzy. Part of our aim in writing this book is to encourage readers to develop further the insights—both statistically and in the various subject areas from which the data come—that can be gained by thinking about appropriate data from a functional point of view. Our own view about what is distinctive about functional data analysis should be gained primarily from the case studies we discuss, as summarized in Section 1.3, but some specific remarks are made in Section 1.4 below.

1.2   The Web site

Working through examples for oneself leads to deeper insight, and is an excellent way into applying and adapting methods to one's own data. To help this process, there is a Web site associated with the text. The Web site contains many of the data sets and analyses discussed in the book. These analyses are *not* intended as a package or as a "cookbook", but our hope is that they will help readers follow the steps that we went through in carrying out the analyses presented in the case studies. Some of the analyses were carried out in MATLAB and some in S-PLUS.

At the time of printing the Web site is linked to the Springer Web site at `www.springer-ny.com`.

1.3   The case studies

In this section, the case studies are briefly reviewed. Further details of the context of the data sets, and appropriate bibliographic references, are given in the individual chapters where the case studies are considered in full. In most of them, in addition to the topics explicitly mentioned below, there is some discussion of computational issues and other fine points of

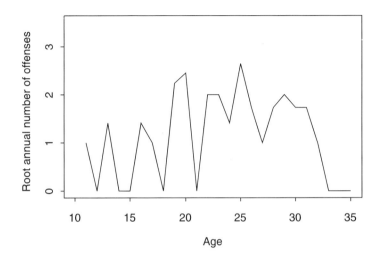

Figure 1.1. The functional datum corresponding to a particular individual in the criminology sample; it shows the way that the annual square root number of crimes varies over the life course.

methodology. In some chapters, we develop or explain some material that will be mainly of interest to statistical experts. These topics are set out in sections towards the end of the relevant chapter, and can be safely skipped by the more general reader.

Chapter 2: Life course data in criminology

We study data on the criminal careers of over 400 individuals followed over several decades of their lifespan. For each individual a function is constructed over the interval $[11, 35]$, representing that person's level of criminal activity between ages 11 and 35. For reasons that are explained, it is appropriate to track the square root of the number of crimes committed each year, and a typical record is given in Figure 1.1. Altogether we consider 413 records like this one, and the records are all plotted in Figure 1.2. This figure demonstrates little more than the need for careful methods of summarizing and analyzing collections of functional data.

Data of this kind are the simplest kind of functional data: we have a number of independent individuals, for each of whom we observe a single function. In standard statistics, we are accustomed to the notion of a sequence of independent numerical observations. This is the functional equivalent: a sequence of independent *functional* observations.

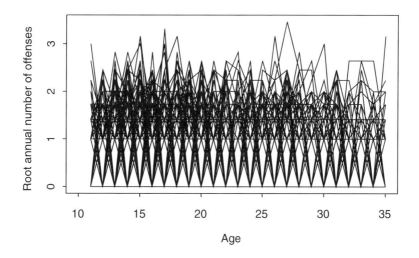

Figure 1.2. The functional data for all 413 subjects in the criminology study.

The questions we address in Chapter 2 include the following.

- What are the steps involved in making raw data on an individual's criminal record into a continuous functional observation?

- How should we estimate the mean of a population such as that in Figure 1.2, and how can we investigate its variability?

- Are there distinct groups of offenders, or do criminals reside on more of a continuum?

- How does our analysis point to salient features of particular data? Of particular interest to criminologists are those individuals who are juvenile offenders who subsequently mature into reasonably law-abiding citizens.

The answers to the third and fourth questions address controversial issues in criminology; it is of obvious importance if there is a "criminal fraternity" with a distinct pattern of offending, and it is also important to know whether reform of young offenders is possible. Quantifying reform is a key step towards this goal.

Chapter 3: The nondurable goods index

In Chapter 3 we turn to a single economic series observed over a long period of time, the U.S. index of nondurable goods production, as plotted

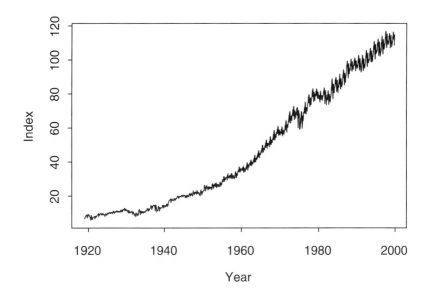

Figure 1.3. The nondurable goods index over the period 1919 to 2000.

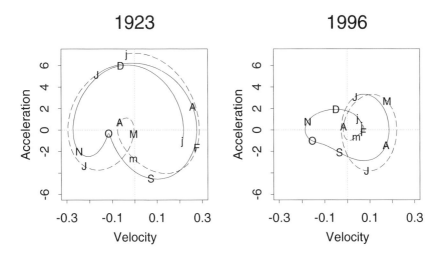

Figure 1.4. Phase-plane plots for two contrasting years: left 1923, right 1996.

in Figure 1.3. Although the index is only produced at monthly intervals, we can think of it as a continuously observed functional time series, with a numerical value at every point over a period of nearly a century. The record for each year may be thought of as an individual functional datum, although of course the point at which each such datum joins to the next is arbitrary; in our analysis, we take it to be the turn of the calendar year.

Our main concern is not the overall level of production, but an investigation of the dynamics of the index within individual years. It is obvious to everyone that goods production nowadays is higher than it was in the 1920s, but more interesting are structural changes in the economy that have affected the detailed behavior, as well as the overall level of activity, over the last century. We pay particular attention to a construct called the *phase-plane plot*, which plots the acceleration of the index against its rate of growth. Figure 1.4 shows phase-plane plots for 1923 and 1996, years near each end of the range of our data.

Our ability to construct phase-plane plots at all depends on the possibility of *differentiating* functional data. In Chapter 3, we use derivatives to construct useful presentations, but in later chapters we take the use of derivatives further, to build and estimate models for the observed functional phenomena.

Chapter 4: Bone shapes from a paleopathology study

Paleopathology is the study of disease in human history, especially taking account of information that can be gathered from human skeletal remains. The study described in Chapter 4 investigates the shapes of a large sample of bones from hundreds of years ago. The intention is to gain knowledge about osteoarthritis of the knee—not just in the past, but nowadays too, because features can be seen that are not easily accessible in living patients. There is evidence of a causal link between the shape of the joint and the incidence of arthritis, and there are plausible biomechanical mechanisms for this link.

We concentrate on images of the knee end of the femur (the upper leg bone); a typical observed shape is shown in Figure 1.5. The functional data considered in Chapter 4 are the outline shapes of bones like this one, and are cyclic curves, not just simple functions of one variable. It is appropriate to characterize these by the positions of *landmarks*. These are specific points picked out on the shapes, and may or may not be of direct interest in themselves.

Specifying landmarks allows a sensible definition of an average bone shape. It also facilitates the investigation of variability in the population, via methods drawn from conventional statistics but with some original twists. Our functional motivation leads to appropriate ways of displaying this variability, and we are able to draw out differences between the bones that show symptoms of arthritis and those that do not.

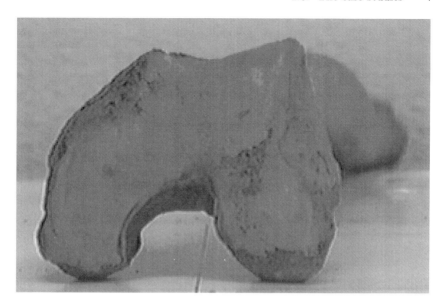

Figure 1.5. A typical raw digital image of a femur from the paleopathology study.

Chapter 5: Modeling reaction time distributions

Attention deficit hyperactive disorder (ADHD) is a troubling condition, especially in children, but is in reality not easily characterized or diagnosed. One important factor may be the reaction time after a visual stimulus. Children that have difficulty in holding attention have slower reaction times than those that can concentrate more easily on a task in hand.

Reaction times are not fixed, but can be thought of as following a distribution specific to each individual. For each child in a study, a sample of about 70 reaction times was collected, and hence an estimate obtained of that child's density function of reaction time. Figure 1.6 shows typical estimated densities, one for an ADHD child and one for a control.

By estimating these densities we have constructed a set of functional data, one curve for each child in the sample. To avoid the difficulties caused by the constraints that probability densities have to obey, and to highlight features of particular relevance, we actually work with the functions obtained by taking logarithms of the densities and differentiating; one aspect of this transformation is that it makes a normal density into a straight line.

Investigating these functional data demonstrates that the difference between the ADHD and control children is not simply an increase in the mean reaction time, but is a more subtle change in the shape of the reaction time distribution.

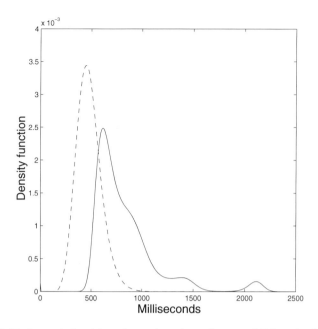

Figure 1.6. Estimated densities of reaction times for two children in the sample. The solid curve corresponds to a child with ADHD, and the dashed curve is one of the controls.

Chapter 6: Zooming in on human growth

Human growth is not at all the simple process that one might imagine at first sight—or even from one's own personal experience of growing up! Studies observing carefully the pattern of growth through childhood and adolescence have been carried out for many decades. A typical data record is shown in Figure 1.7. Collecting records like these is time-consuming and expensive, because children have to be measured accurately and tracked for a long period of their lives.

We consider how to make this sort of record into a useful functional datum to incorporate into further analyses. A smooth curve drawn through the points in Figure 1.7 is commonly called a growth curve, but growth is actually the *rate of increase* of the height of the child. In children this is necessarily positive because it is only much later in life that people begin to lose stature. We develop a monotone smoothing method that takes this sort of consideration into account and yields a functional datum that picks out important stages in a child's growth.

Not all children go through events such as puberty at the same age. Once the functional data have been obtained, an important issue is time-warping or *registration*. Here the aim is to refer all the children to a common biological clock. Only then is it really meaningful to talk about a mean growth pattern or to investigate variability in the sample. Also, the relationship of

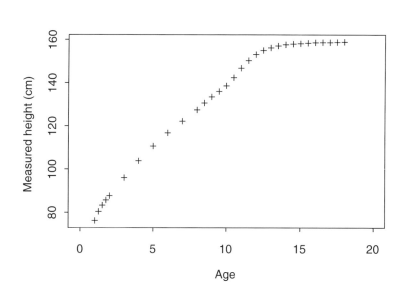

Figure 1.7. The raw data for a particular individual in a classical growth study.

biological to chronological age is itself important, and can also be seen as an interesting functional datum for each child.

The monotone smoothing method also allows the consideration of data observed on much shorter time scales than those in Figure 1.7. The results are fascinating, demonstrating that growth does not occur smoothly, but consists of short bursts of rapid growth interspersed by periods of relative stability. The length and spacing of these *saltations* can be very short, especially in babies, where our results suggest growth cycles of length just a few days.

Chapter 7: Time warping handwriting and weather records

In much biomechanical research nowadays, electronic tracking equipment is used to track body movements in real time as certain tasks are performed. One of us wrote the characters "fda" 20 times, and the resulting pen traces are shown in Figure 1.8. But the data we are actually able to work with are the full trace in time of all three coordinates of the pen position.

To study the important features of these curves, time registration is essential. We use this case study to develop more fully the ideas of registration introduced in Chapter 6, and we discover that there are dynamic patterns that become much more apparent once we refer to an appropriate time scale.

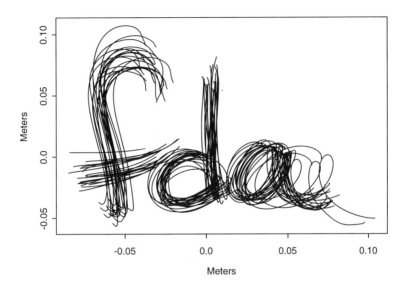

Figure 1.8. The characters "fda" written by hand 20 times.

Weather records are a rich source of functional data, as variables such as temperature and pressure are recorded through time. We know from our own experience that the seasons do not always fall at exactly the same calendar date, and one of the effects of global climate change may be disruption in the annual cycle as much as in the actual temperatures achieved. Both *phase variation*, the variability in the time warping function, and *amplitude variation*, the variability in the actual curve values, are important. This study provides an opportunity to explain how these aspects of variability can be separated, and to explore some consequences for the analysis of weather data.

Chapter 8: How do bone shapes indicate arthritis?

Here we return to the bones considered in Chapter 4, and focus attention on the *intercondylar notch*, the inverted U-shape between the two ends of the bone as displayed in Figure 1.5. There are anatomical reasons why the shape of the intercondylar notch may be especially relevant to the incidence of arthritis. In addition, some of the bones are damaged in ways that exclude them from the analysis described in Chapter 4, but do not affect the intercondylar notch.

The landmark methods used when considering the entire cyclical shape are not easily applicable. Therefore we develop landmark-free approaches to the functional data analysis of curves, such as the notch outlines, traced out in two (or more) dimensions. Once these curves are represented in an appropriate way, it becomes possible to analyze different modes of variability in the data.

Of particular interest is a functional analogue of *linear discriminant analysis*. If we wanted to find out a way of distinguishing arthritic and nonarthritic intercondylar notch shapes, simply finding the mean shape within each group is not a very good way to go. On the other hand, blindly applying discriminant methods borrowed from standard multivariate analysis gives nonsensical results. By incorporating *regularization* in the right way, however, we can find a mode of variability that is good at separating the two kinds of bones. What seems to matter is the twist in the shape of the notch, which may well affect the way that an important ligament lies in the joint.

Chapter 9: Functional models for test items

Now we move from the way our ancestors walked to the way our children are tested in school. Perhaps surprisingly, functional data analysis ideas can bring important insights to the way that different test questions work in practice. Assume for the moment that we have a one-dimensional abstract measure θ of ability. For question i we can then define the *item response function* $P_i(\theta)$ to be the probability that a candidate of ability θ answers this question correctly.

The particular case study concentrates on the performance of 5000 candidates on 60 questions in a test constructed by the American College Testing Program. Some of the steps in our analysis are the following.

- There is no explicit definition of ability θ, but we construct a suitable θ from the data, and estimate the individual item response functions $P_i(\theta)$.

- By considering the estimated item response functions as functional data in their own right, we identify important aspects of the test questions, both as a sample and individually. Both graphical and more analytical methods are used.

- We investigate important questions raised by splitting the sample into female and male candidates. Can ability be assessed in a gender-neutral way? Are there questions on which men and women perform differently? There are only a few such test items in our data, but results for two of them are plotted in Figure 1.9. Which of these questions you would find easier would depend both on your gender and on your position on the overall ability range as quantified by the estimated score θ.

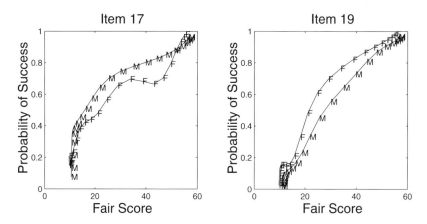

Figure 1.9. Probabilities of success on two test questions are displayed for both females and males, against a fair score that is a reasonable gender-neutral measure of ability.

Chapter 10: Predicting lip acceleration from electromyography

Over 100 muscles are involved in speech, and our ability to control and coordinate them is remarkable. The limitation on the rate of production of phonemes—perhaps 14 per second—is cognitive rather than physical. If we were designing a system for controlling speech movements, we would plan sequences of movements as a group, rather than simply executing each movement as it came along. Does the brain do this?

This big question can be approached by studying the movement of the lower lip during speech and taking electromyography (EMG) recordings to detect associated neural activity. The lower lip is an obvious subset of muscles to concentrate on because it is easily observed and the EMG recordings can be taken from skin surface electrodes. The larynx would offer neither advantage!

A subject is observed repeatedly saying a particular phrase. After preprocessing, smoothing, and registration, this yields paired functional observations $(Y_i(t), Z_i(t))$, where Y_i is the lip acceleration and Z_i is the EMG level. If the brain just does things on the fly, then these data could be modeled by the pointwise model

$$Y_i(t) = \alpha(t) + Z_i(t)\beta(t) + \epsilon_i(t). \tag{1.1}$$

On the other hand, if there is feedforward information for a period of length δ in the neural control mechanism, then a model of the form

$$Y_i(t) = \alpha(t) + \int_{t-\delta}^{t} Z_i(s)\beta(s,t)\,ds + \epsilon_i(t) \tag{1.2}$$

may be more appropriate.

The study investigates aspects of these formulations of *functional linear regression*. The EMG functions play the role of the independent variable and the lip accelerations that of the dependent variable. Because of the functional nature of both, there is a choice of the structure of the model to fit. For the particular data studied, the indication is that there is indeed feedforward information, especially in certain parts of the articulated phrase.

Chapter 11: The dynamics of handwriting printed characters

The subject of this study is handwriting data as exemplified in Figure 1.8. Generally, we are used to identifying people we know well by their handwriting. Since in this case we have dynamic data about the way the pen actually moved during the writing, even including the periods it is off the paper, we might expect to be able to do better still.

It turns out that the X-, Y-, and Z-coordinates of data of this kind can all be modeled remarkably closely by a linear differential equation model of the form

$$u'''(t) = \alpha(t) + \beta_1(t)u'(t) + \beta_2(t)u''(t). \qquad (1.3)$$

The coefficient functions $\alpha(t)$, $\beta_1(t)$, and $\beta_2(t)$ depend on which coordinate of the writing one is considering, and are specific to the writer. In this study, we investigate the ways that models of this kind can be fitted to data using a method called *principal differential analysis*.

The principal differential analysis of a particular person's handwriting gives some insight into the biomechanical processes underlying handwriting. In addition, we show that the fitted model is good at the classification problem of deciding who wrote what. You may well be able to forge the shape of someone else's signature, but you will have difficulty in producing a pen trace in real time that satisfies that person's differential equation model.

Chapter 12: A differential equation for juggling

Nearly all readers will be good at handwriting, but not many will be equally expert jugglers. An exception is statistician Michael Newton at Wisconsin, and data observed from Michael's juggling are the subject of our final case study. Certainly to less talented mortals, there is an obvious difference between handwriting and juggling: when we write, the paper remains still and we are always trying to do the same thing; a juggler seems to be catching and throwing balls that all follow different paths.

Various markers on Michael's body were tracked, but we concentrate on the tip of his forefinger. The juggling cycles are not of constant length, because if the ball is thrown higher it takes longer to come back down, and so there is some preprocessing to be done. After this has been achieved, the

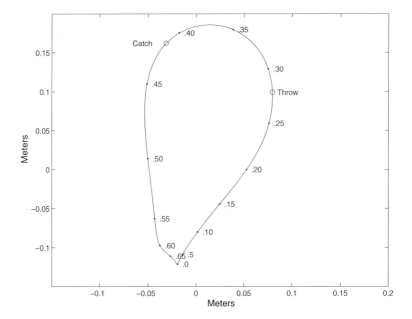

Figure 1.10. The average juggling cycle as seen from the juggler's perspective facing forward. The points on the curve indicate times in seconds, and the total cycle takes 0.711 seconds. The time when the ball leaves the hand and the time of the catch are shown as circles.

average juggling cycle is shown from one view in Figure 1.10. More details are given in Chapter 12.

Although individual cycles vary, they can all be modeled closely by a differential equation approach building on that of Chapter 11. There is a key difference, however; for the handwriting data the model (1.3) was used to model each coordinate separately. In juggling, there is crosstalk between the coordinates, with the derivatives and second derivatives of some affecting the third derivatives of others. However, there is no need for the terms corresponding to $\alpha(t)$ in the model.

Various aspects of the coordinate functions $\beta(t)$ are discussed. Most interestingly, the resulting system of differential equations controls all the individual juggling cycles almost perfectly, despite the outward differences among the cycles. Learning to juggle almost corresponds to wiring the system of differential equations into one's brain and motor system.

1.4   How is functional data analysis distinctive?

The actual term *functional data analysis* was coined by Ramsay and Dalzell (1991), although many of the ideas have of course been around for much longer in some form. What has been more distinctive about recent research is the notion of functional data analysis as a unified way of thinking, rather than a disparate set of methods and techniques.

We have quite deliberately refrained from attempting an exhaustive definition of functional data analysis, because we do not wish to set hard boundaries around the field. Nevertheless, it may be worth noting some common aspects of functional data that arise frequently in this book and elsewhere.

- *Conceptually, functional data are continuously defined.* Of course, in practice they are usually observed at discrete points and also have to be stored in some finite-dimensional way within the computer, but this does not alter our underlying way of thinking.

- *The individual datum is the whole function*, rather than its value at any particular point. The various functional data will often be independent of one another, but there are no particular assumptions about the independence of different values within the same functional datum.

- In some cases the data are functions of time, but *there is nothing special about time as a variable.* In the case studies we have been involved in, the data are functions of a one-dimensional variable, but most of the insights carry over straightforwardly to functions of higher-dimensional variables.

- There is no general requirement that the data be smooth, but *often smoothness or other regularity will be a key aspect of the analysis.* In some cases, derivatives of the observed functions will be important. On other occasions, even though the data themselves need not be smooth, smoothness assumptions will be appropriate for mean functions or other functions involved in modeling the observed data.

1.5   Conclusion and bibliography

Those wishing to read further are referred initially to the book by Ramsay and Silverman (1997), which gives a thematic treatment of many of the topics introduced by case studies in the present volume. That book also contains many additional bibliographic references and technical details. Of particular relevance to this introduction are Chapters 1 and 16 of Ramsay and Silverman (1997). These both stand aside somewhat from specific methods but discuss the general philosophy of functional data analysis. Chapter 16, in particular, considers the historical context of the subject as well as raising some issues for further investigation. Many of the case studies presented in this book are the fruits of our own continuing research in response to this challenge. Although our present book approaches functional data analysis from a different direction, the remark (Ramsay and Silverman, 1997, page 21) made in our previous book remains equally true:

> In broad terms, we have a grander aim: to encourage readers to think about and understand functional data in a new way. The methods we set out are hardly the last word in approaching the particular problems, and we believe that readers will gain more benefit by using the principles we have laid down than by following our suggestions to the letter.

Even more than a thematic treatment, case studies will always lead the alert reader to suggest and investigate approaches that are different, and perhaps better, than those originally presented. If a reader is prompted by one of our chapters to find a better way of dealing with a functional data set, then our aim of encouraging further functional data analysis research and development will certainly have been fulfilled.

2
Life Course Data in Criminology

2.1 Criminology life course studies

2.1.1 Background

An important question in criminology is the study of the way that people's level of criminal activity varies through their lives. Can it be said that there are "career criminals" of different kinds? Are there particular patterns of persistence in the levels of crimes committed by individuals? These issues have been studied by criminologists for many years. Of continuing importance is the question of whether there are distinct subgroups or clusters within the population, or whether observed criminal behaviors are part of a continuum. Naturally, one pattern of particular interest is "desistance', the discontinuation of regular offending.

The classic study Glueck and Glueck (1950) considered the criminal histories of 500 delinquent boys. The Gluecks and subsequent researchers (especially Sampson and Laub, 1993) carried out a prospective longitudinal study of the formation and development of criminal "careers" of the individuals in their sample. The subjects were initially interviewed at age around 14, and were followed up subsequently, both by personal interview and through FBI and police records. The main part of the data was collected by the Gluecks themselves over the period 1940 to 1965, but there are subsequent data right up to the present day, giving individual life course information up to age 70. These data are very unusual in providing long-term longitudinal information; most criminological data are cross-sectional or at best longitudinal only over restricted age ranges.

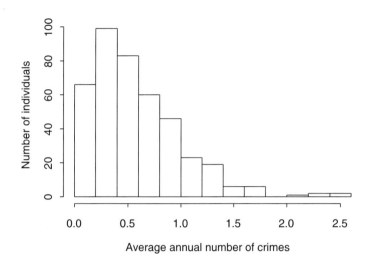

Figure 2.1. Histogram of the average annual number of arrests for each of 413 men over a 25-year time period.

The objective is to understand the pattern or trajectory through life of offending for the members of the sample. For each individual, the number of official arrests in each year of their life is recorded, starting in some cases as early as age 7. Obviously these are only a surrogate for the number of crimes committed, but they give a good indication of the general level of criminal activity. There is information on the type of crime and also on various concomitant information, but we do not consider this in detail.

2.1.2   The life course data

We concentrate on a single set of data giving the numbers of arrests of 413 men over a 25-year period in each of their lives, from age 11 to age 35. These are the individuals for whom we have full information over this period. An immediate indication of the diversity within the group is given by considering the overall annual average number of arrests for each individual. Figure 2.1 shows that some of the men had only a low overall arrest rate, while others were clearly habitual offenders with 50 or more arrests registered in total. It is also clear that the distribution is highly skewed.

Another aspect is the high variability for each individual over time. Figure 2.2 shows the raw data for a typical individual. It can be seen that this person was arrested in connection with three offenses at age 11, one at age 14, and so on. The small numbers of crimes each year mean that

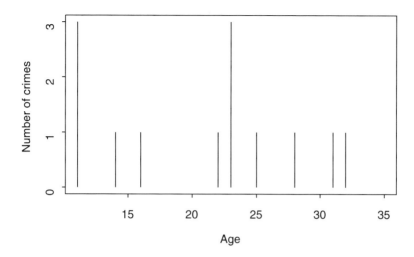

Figure 2.2. The record of a particular individual, showing the numbers of arrests at various ages. This individual was arrested for three offenses at age 11, one at age 14, and so on, but was not arrested at all in years 12, 13, 15, etc.

every individual is likely to show a sporadic pattern of some sort. Despite the very noisy nature of the data, one of our aims is to find ways of quantifying meaningful patterns in individuals that reflect variation in the wider population.

Our analysis raises a number of questions of broader importance in functional data analysis. The approach is to represent the criminal record of each subject by a single function of time, and then to use these functions for detailed analysis. But how should discrete observations be made into functional data in the first place? Does the functional nature of the data have any implications when producing smoothed estimates of quantities such as the overall mean curve? How can meaningful aspects of variation of the entire population be estimated and quantified in the presence of such large variability in individuals?

2.2 First steps in a functional approach

2.2.1 Turning discrete values into a functional datum

We construct for each individual a function of time that represents his level of criminal activity. A simple approach would be to interpolate the raw

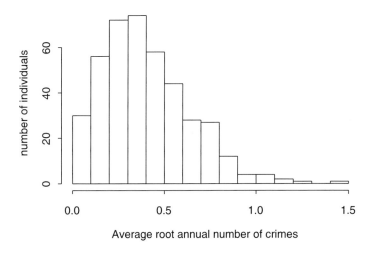

Figure 2.3. Histogram of the averages for each of 413 individuals of the square roots of annual tallies of arrests.

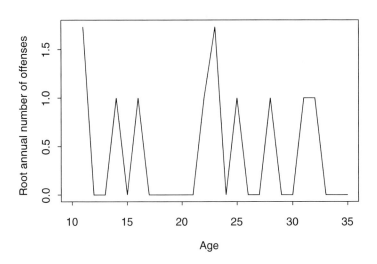

Figure 2.4. Linear interpolant of the square roots of the counts shown in Figure 2.2.

numbers of arrests in each year, but because of the skewness of the annual counts this would give inordinate weight to high values in the original data. In order to stabilize the variability somewhat, we start by taking the square root of the number of arrests each year. The rationale for this is partly pragmatic: if we plot a histogram of the averages across time of these square roots we see from Figure 2.3 that the skewness is somewhat reduced. In addition, if the numbers of arrests are Poisson counts, then the square root is the standard variance-stabilizing transformation.

One could conceivably smooth the square roots of annual counts to produce a functional observation for the individual considered in Figure 2.2. However, in order not to suppress any information at this stage, we interpolate linearly to produce the functional observation shown in Figure 2.4. We now throw away the original points and regard this function as a whole as being the datum for this individual. In the remainder of this chapter, we denote by $Y_1(t), Y_2(t), \ldots, Y_{413}(t)$ the 413 functional observations constructed from the square roots of the annual arrest count for the 413 individuals in the study.

2.2.2 Estimating the mean

The next step in the analysis of the data is to estimate the mean function of the functional data. The natural estimator to begin with is simply the sample average defined in this case by

$$\bar{Y}(t) = \frac{1}{413} \sum_{i=1}^{413} Y_i(t).$$

The function $\bar{Y}(t)$ is plotted in Figure 2.5. It can be seen that, despite the large number of functions on which the mean is based, there is still some fluctuation in the result of a kind that is clearly not relevant to the problem at hand; there is no reason why 29-year olds commit fewer offenses than both 28- and 30-year olds for instance! Before embarking on a discussion of smoothing the mean function, it should be pointed out that this particular set of data has high local variability. In many other practical examples no smoothing will be necessary.

There are many possible approaches to the smoothing of the curve in Figure 2.5, and the one we use is a *roughness penalty* method. We measure the roughness, or variability, of a curve g by the integrated squared second derivative of g. Our estimate of the overall mean is then the curve $m_\lambda(t)$ that minimizes the penalized squared error

$$S_\lambda(g) = \int \{g(t) - \bar{Y}(t)\}^2 dt + \lambda \int \{g''(t)\}^2 dt. \qquad (2.1)$$

Here the *smoothing parameter* $\lambda \geq 0$ controls the trade-off between closeness of fit to the average of the data, as measured by the first integral in

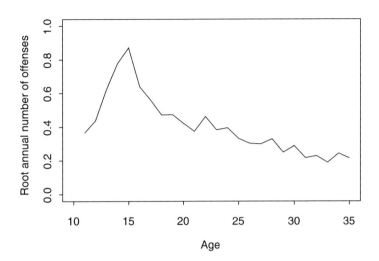

Figure 2.5. The sample mean function of the criminology functional data.

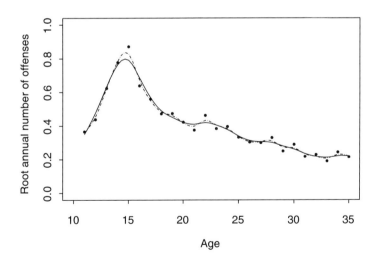

Figure 2.6. Estimate of the overall mean of the square root of the number of arrests per year. Points: raw means of the data. Dashed curve: roughness penalty smooth, $\lambda = 2 \times 10^{-7}$, cross-validation choice. Solid curve: roughness penalty smooth, $\lambda = 10^{-6}$, subjective adjustment.

(2.1) and the variability of the curve, as measured by the second integral. Both integrals are taken over the range of the parameter t, in this case from 11 to 35. If $\lambda = 0$ then the curve $m_\lambda(t)$ is equal to the sample mean curve $\bar{Y}(t)$. As λ increases, the curve $m_\lambda(t)$ gets closer to the standard linear regression fit to the values of $\bar{Y}(t)$.

In practice, the smoothing parameter λ has to be chosen to obtain a curve $m_\lambda(t)$ that is reasonably faithful to the original sample average but eliminates obviously extraneous variability. In practice, it is often easiest to choose the smoothing parameter subjectively, but in some circumstances an automatic choice of smoothing parameter may be useful, if only as a starting point for further subjective adjustment. An approach to this automatic choice using a method called *cross-validation* is discussed in Section 2.6. In Figure 2.6 we give the smoothed mean curve obtained by an automatic choice of smoothing, and also the effect of a subjective adjustment to this automatic choice. For the remainder of our analysis, this subjectively smoothed curve is used as an estimate of the overall mean function. We use the subjectively smoothed curve rather than the initial automatic choice because of the need to have a firm stable reference curve against which to judge individuals later in the analysis. In constructing this reference, we want to be sure that spurious variability is kept to a minimum.

2.3   Functional principal component analyses

2.3.1   The basic methodology

What are the types of variability between the boys in the sample? There is controversy among criminologists as to whether there are distinct criminal groups or types. Some maintain that there are, for instance, specific groups of high offenders, or persistent offenders. Others reject this notion and consider that there is a continuum of levels and types of offending.

Principal components analysis (PCA) is a standard approach to the exploration of variability in multivariate data. PCA uses an eigenvalue decomposition of the variance matrix of the data to find directions in the observation space along which the data have the highest variability. For each principal component, the analysis yields a *loading vector* or *weight vector* which gives the direction of variability corresponding to that component. For details, see any standard multivariate analysis textbook, such as Johnson and Wichern (2002).

In the functional context, each principal component is specified by a *principal component weight function* $\xi(t)$ defined over the same range of t as the functional data. The principal component scores of the individuals in the sample are the values z_i given by

$$z_i = \int \xi(t)Y_i(t)dt. \tag{2.2}$$

The aim of simple PCA is to find the weight function $\xi_1(t)$ that maximizes the variance of the principal component scores z_i subject to the constraint

$$\int \xi(t)^2 dt = 1. \qquad (2.3)$$

Without a constraint of this kind, we could make the variance as large as we liked simply by multiplying ξ by a large quantity.

The second-, third-, and higher-order principal components are defined in the same way, but with additional constraints. The second component function $\xi_2(t)$ is defined to maximize the variance of the principal component scores subject to the constraint (2.3) and the additional constraint

$$\int \xi_2(t)\xi_1(t)dt = 0. \qquad (2.4)$$

In general, for the jth component we require the additional constraints

$$\int \xi_j(t)\xi_1(t)dt = \int \xi_j(t)\xi_2(t)dt = \ldots = \int \xi_j(t)\xi_{j-1}(t) = 0, \qquad (2.5)$$

which will ensure that all the estimated principal components are mutually orthogonal.

In the case of the criminology data, the approach just described corresponds approximately to the following; the approximation is due to the approximation of the integrals by sums in (2.2) through (2.5).

1. Regard each of the functional data as a vector in 25-dimensional space, by reading off the values at each year of the individual's age.

2. Carry out a standard PCA on the resulting data set of 413 observations in 25-dimensional space.

3. Interpolate each principal component weight vector to give a weight function.

In Figure 2.7 the results of this approach are illustrated. For each of the first three principal components, three curves are plotted. The dashed curve is the overall smoothed mean, which is the same in all cases. The other two curves show the effect of adding and subtracting a suitable multiple of the principal component weight function.

It can be seen that the first principal component corresponds to the overall level of offending from about age 15 to age 35. All the components have a considerable amount of local variability, and in the case of the second component, particularly, this almost overwhelms any systematic effect. Clearly some smoothing is appropriate, not surprisingly given the high variability of the data.

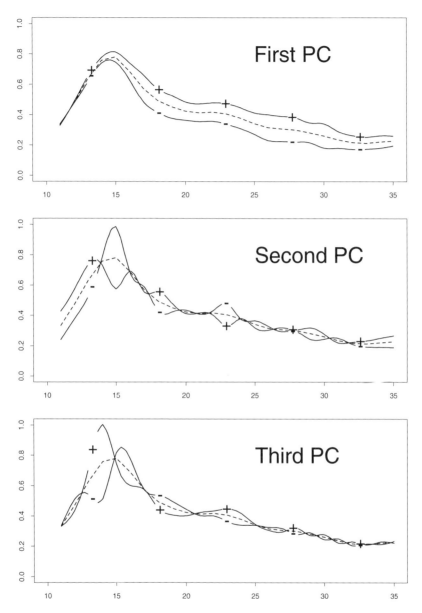

Figure 2.7. The effect of the first three unsmoothed principal components of the criminology data. In each graph, the dashed curve is the overall mean, and the solid curves are the mean ± a suitable multiple of the relevant principal component weight function. The + and − signs show which curve is which.

2.3.2 Smoothing the PCA

Smoothing a functional principal component analysis is not just a matter of smoothing the components produced by a standard PCA. Rather, we return to the original definition of principal components analysis and incorporate smoothing into that. Let us consider the leading principal component first of all.

To obtain a smoothed functional PCA, we take account of the need not only to control the size of ξ, but also to control its roughness. With this in mind, we replace the constraint (2.3) by a constraint that takes roughness into account as well. Thus, the first smoothed principal component weight function is the function $\xi_1(t)$ that maximizes the variance of the principal component scores subject to the constraint

$$\int \{\xi(t)\}^2 dt + \alpha \int \{\xi''(t)\}^2 dt = 1. \qquad (2.6)$$

As usual, the parameter $\alpha \geq 0$ controls the amount of smoothing inherent in the procedure.

A roughness penalty is also incorporated into the additional constraints on the second-, third-, and higher-order smoothed principal components. The second component function $\xi_2(t)$ is now defined to maximize the variance of the principal component scores subject to (2.6) and the additional constraint

$$\int \xi_2(t)\xi_1(t)dt + \alpha \int \xi_2''(t)\xi_1''(t)dt = 0. \qquad (2.7)$$

For the jth component we require constraints analogous to (2.5), but with corresponding extra terms taking the roughness penalty into account. This will ensure that the estimated components satisfy the condition

$$\int \xi_i(t)\xi_j(t)dt + \alpha \int \xi_i''(t)\xi_j''(t)dt = 0$$

for all i and j with $i \neq j$.

There are some attractive features to this approach to defining a smoothed principal components analysis. First, when $\alpha = 0$, we recover the standard unsmoothed PCA of the data. Second, despite the recursive nature of their definition, the principal components can be found in a single linear algebra calculation; details are given in Section 2.5.3.

2.3.3 Smoothed PCA of the criminology data

The first three principal component weight functions arising from a smoothed PCA are given in Figure 2.8. The smoothing parameter was chosen by subjective adjustment to the value $\alpha = 10^{-5}$. It can be seen that each of these components now has a clear interpretation.

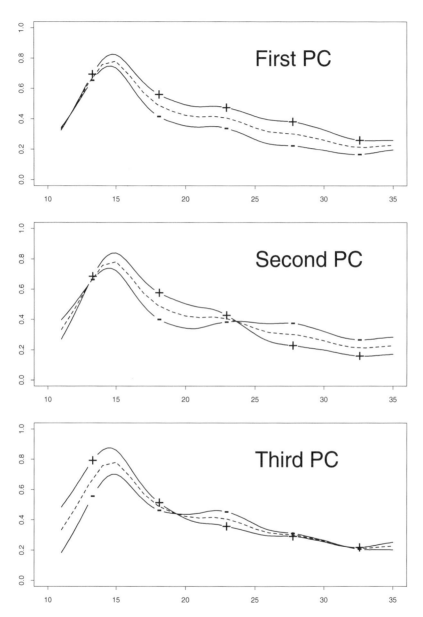

Figure 2.8. The effect on the mean curve of adding and subtracting a multiple of each of the first three smoothed functional principal components. The smoothing parameter was set to $\alpha = 10^{-5}$.

The first quantifies the general level of criminal activity throughout later adolescence and adulthood. A high scorer on this component would show especially above-average activity in the years from age 18 to age 30. It is interesting that this increased difference is not in the teenage years when the general level is very high anyway. High scorers on this component are above average during late adolescence but not markedly so; it is in their late teens and twenties that they depart most strongly from the mean. For this reason we call this component "Adult crime level."

The second component indicates a mode of variability corresponding to high activity up to the early twenties, then reforming to better than average in later years. High scorers are juvenile delinquents who then see the error of their ways and reform permanently. On the other hand those with large negative scores are well-behaved teenagers who then later take up a life of crime. We call this component "Long-term desistance."

The third component measures activity earlier in life. High scorers on this component are high offenders right from childhood through their teenage years. The component then shows a bounceback in the early twenties, later reverting to overall average behavior. This component is most affected by juvenile criminal activity and we call it "Juvenile crime level."

Sampson and Laub (1993, Chapter 1) place particular emphasis on early onset of delinquency and on adult desistance as important aspects of the life course often neglected by criminologists. Our analysis supports their claim, because the smoothed principal components analysis has picked out components corresponding to these features.

2.3.4   Detailed examination of the scores

We now find the score of each of the 413 individuals in the sample on these three principal components, by integrating the weight function against the functional datum in each case. This gives each individual a score on each of the attributes "adult," "desistance," and "juvenile." These are plotted in pairs in Figure 2.9. There is essentially no correlation among these scores, so the three aspects can be considered as uncorrelated within the population.

However, the distribution of the first component, labeled "Adult" in the plots, is very skewed, with a long tail to the right; note that the mean of these scores is only 1.8. Even after taking the square root transformation, there are some individuals with very high overall rates of offending. If the overall score is low, then the values of "Desistance" are tightly clustered, but this is not the case for higher levels. This is for the simple reason that individuals with low overall crime rates have no real scope either to desist strongly, or to increase strongly. Because the overall rate cannot be negative, there are, essentially, constraints on the size of the second component in terms of that of the first, and these are visible in the plot. What the plot shows is that individuals with high overall rates can equally

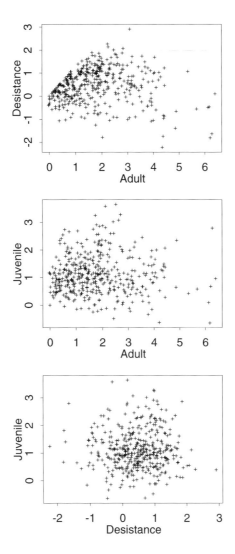

Figure 2.9. Plots of the first three principal components scores of the criminology life course data. The mean of the Adult scores is about 1.8.

well be strong desisters or strong "late developers." The same variability of behavior is not possible among low offenders.

The second and third components have symmetric unimodal distributions, and the third plot gives the kind of scatter one would expect from an uncorrelated bivariate normal distribution. The second plot of course shows the skewness of the "Adult" variable, but otherwise shows no very distinctive features.

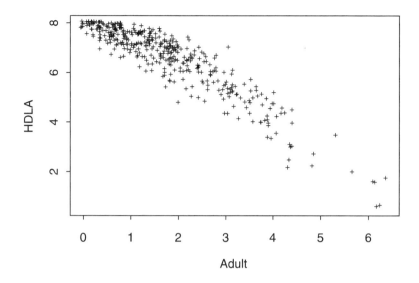

Figure 2.10. High desistance/low adult score plotted against Adult score.

Let us return to the plot of Adult against Desistance scores. An important issue in criminology is the existence of distinct groups of individuals in the population. There is no suggestion in this plot of a cluster of high-crime individuals even though there is a long tail in the distribution. However, there does appear to be a preponderance of cases near the upper boundary of the plotted points toward the left of the picture. These are all individuals with low adult crime rates and with nearly the maximum possible desistance for their adult crime scores. In order to identify these cases, we introduce a high desistance/low adult (HDLA) score, defined by

$$HDLA = 0.7 \times (\text{Desistance score}) - (\text{Adult score}) + 8.$$

A plot of the HDLA score against the Adult score is given in Figure 2.10. The multiple of 0.7 in the definition of HDLA was chosen to make the boundary at the top of this plot horizontal. The arbitrary constant 8 was added to make all the scores positive. We can see that there is a range of values of Adult scores for which HDLA is near its maximum value. A histogram of the HDLA values is given in Figure 2.11. Although the individuals with HDLA values near the maximum do not form a separate group, there is certainly a strong tendency for a cluster to form near this value. What do the trajectories of such individuals look like?

Ignoring all other variability, we examine the raw data of the 36 individuals with HDLA scores above 7.87. These are plotted in Figure 2.12. The individual trajectories cannot be easily distinguished, but the message

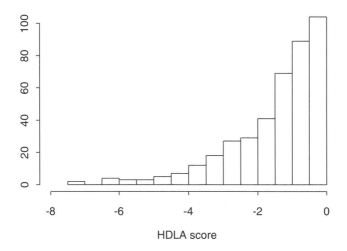

Figure 2.11. Histogram of the HDLA scores.

is clear: these are individuals who give up crime altogether by their late teens, even though earlier on they may have been quite high offenders. This is confirmed by Figure 2.13, which compares the HDLA score to the last age at which any offense is committed. A small number of individuals have very high HDLA scores but still offend very sporadically later in life. Thus the HDLA score is a more robust measure of almost total desistance than is the simple statistic of the last age at which any offense is committed.

2.4   What have we seen?

Constructing functional observations from discrete data is not always straightforward, and it is often preferable to transform the original data in some way. In the case of the criminology life course data, a square root of the original annual counts gave good results.

A key feature of the life course data is the high variability of the individual functional data. Even though there are over 400 curves, the sample mean curve still contains noticeable spurious fluctuation. A roughness penalty smoothing approach gives a natural way of incorporating smoothing into the estimation of the mean. In the functional context, some guidance as to the appropriate value of the smoothing parameter can be obtained by a cross-validation method discussed in more detail below.

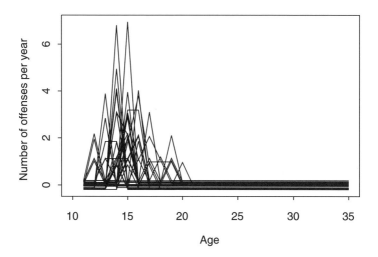

Figure 2.12. Raw data for the individuals with HDLA scores above 0.27. The data have been slightly jittered in order to separate the lines.

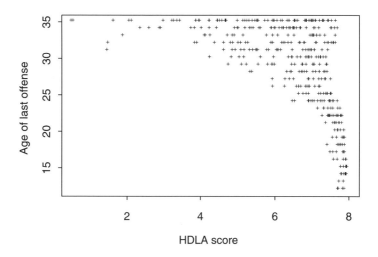

Figure 2.13. Age of last recorded offense plotted against HDLA scores. The individuals with highest HDLA scores correspond closely to those who give up crime altogether by age 20.

Without some smoothing, a functional principal components analysis of these data does not give very meaningful results. However, good results can be obtained by incorporating a roughness penalty into the size constraint of the principal component weight functions. The various principal components have immediate interpretations in terms of the original criminological issues, and can be used to build a composite score, the high desistance/low adult score, which brings out particular features of importance. There is no real evidence of strong grouping within the original data.

At this point, we have finished the specific task of analyzing the criminology data, but our discussion has raised two particular matters that are worth exploring in more detail. A general matter is the way that functional observations are stored and processed. A more specific issue is the cross-validation approach to the choice of smoothing parameter when estimating the mean. Some readers may wish to skip these sections, especially Section 2.5.2 onwards.

2.5 How are functions stored and processed?

2.5.1 Basis expansions

In the example we have considered, we could simply store all the original values at the 25 evaluation points, since these points are the same for each individual in the sample. However, there are several reasons for considering other approaches. First, it is in the spirit of functional data analysis that we wish to specify the whole function, not just its value at a finite number of points. Second, it is important to have a method that can generalize to the case where the evaluation points are not the same for every individual in the sample. Third, we will often wish to be able to evaluate the derivatives of a functional datum or other function we are considering.

A good way of storing functional observations is in terms of a suitable *basis*. A basis is a standard set of functions, denoted $\beta_1(t), \beta_2(t), \ldots, \beta_m(t)$, for example, such that any function of interest can be expanded in terms of the functions $\beta_j(t)$. If a functional datum $x(t)$ is written

$$x(t) = \sum_{j=1}^{m} \xi_j \beta_j(t) \qquad (2.8)$$

then the vector of m coefficients $\xi = (\xi_1, \ldots, \xi_m)$ specifies the function.

Storing functional data in terms of an appropriate basis is a key step in most functional data analyses. Very often, the basis is defined implicitly within the procedure and there is no need for the user to be aware of it. For example, our treatment of the criminology life course data used a very simple basis, the *polygonal basis* made up of triangular functions like the ones shown in Figure 2.14. In mathematical terms, the basis functions $\delta_i(t)$

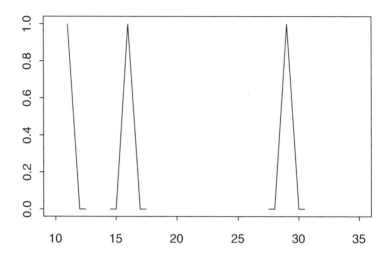

Figure 2.14. Three triangular basis functions. The functions are zero outside the range plotted.

are defined for $i = 1, 2, \ldots, 25$ and $11 \leq t \leq 35$ by setting $t_i = i + 10$ and

$$\delta_i(t) = \begin{cases} 1 - |t - t_i| & \text{if } |t - t_i| < 1 \\ 0 & \text{otherwise.} \end{cases} \tag{2.9}$$

The coefficients ξ_j of a particular function are, in this case, exactly the values $x(j + 10)$ of the function at the evaluation points. In between these points the function is interpolated linearly.

Because the basis functions $\delta_j(t)$ are not themselves everywhere smooth, they will not give rise to smooth basis expansions either. A good basis for the representation of smooth functions is a basis of B-splines, as plotted in Figure 2.15. B-splines are a flexible and numerically stable basis that is very commonly used. Except near the boundaries, the B-splines we use are all identical bell-shaped curves. The nonzero part of each B-spline is a piecewise cubic polynomial, with four cubic pieces fitting together smoothly to give a curve that has jumps only in its third derivative.

In the following sections, we give more details of the calculations involving basis expansions. These are intended for readers who are interested in the way that the basis expansions are used in practice and might wish to reconstruct the calculations for themselves. The algorithms are not explained in detail, but the more mathematically sophisticated reader not willing to take the results on trust should have no difficulty in reconstructing the arguments underlying them.

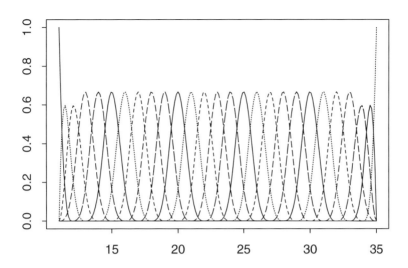

Figure 2.15. A B-spline basis that can be used to represent smooth functions

The first step is to use discrete observations of a function to obtain a basis representation. Then we move to the ways in which the smoothed mean estimation and the smoothed principal components analysis are carried out for a set of functional data held in basis representation form. The life course data are used as a concrete example, but the general principles can be extended widely. Some of this material is discussed in more detail in Ramsay and Silverman (1997) but it is convenient to draw it all together here. Some additional material, including S-PLUS software, is given in the Web page corresponding to this chapter.

2.5.2 Fitting basis coefficients to the observed data

Consider the criminology data for a single individual in the sample. In our case the function corresponding to that individual is specified at the 25 points corresponding to ages from 11 to 35, and a triangular basis is used. More generally we will have values $x_1, x_2, \ldots, x_n$ at n *evaluation points* $t_1, t_2, \ldots, t_n$, and we will have a more general set of basis functions $\beta_j(t)$. Define the $n \times m$ matrix B to have elements

$$B_{ij} = \beta_j(t_i),$$

so that if the coefficient vector is ξ then the vector of values at the evaluation points is $B\xi$.

There are now two cases to consider.[1] If there are no more basis functions than evaluation points, so that $m \leq n$, then we can fit the basis functions by least squares, to minimize the sum of squares of deviations between x_k and $\sum_j \xi_j \beta_j(t_k)$. By standard statistical least squares theory, setting

$$\xi = (B'B)^{-1}B'x$$

will then specify the coefficients completely. If $m = n$ the resulting expansion $x(t) = \sum_j \xi_j \beta_j(t)$ will interpolate the values x_i exactly, whereas if $m < n$ the expansion will be a smoothed version of the original data. In the criminology data example, the matrix B is the identity matrix and so we simply set $\xi = x$.

On the other hand, if there are more basis functions than evaluation points, there will be many choices of ξ that will interpolate the given values exactly, so that

$$x_k = \sum_{j=1}^{m} \xi_j \beta_j(t_k) \text{ for each } k = 1, 2, \ldots, n, \qquad (2.10)$$

which can be written in vector form as $B\xi = x$. In order to choose between these, we choose the parameters that minimize the roughness of the curve, suitably quantified. For instance, if a B-spline basis is used, we can use the roughness penalty $\int \{x''(t)\}^2 dt$. Define the matrix K by

$$K_{ij} = \int \beta_i''(t)\beta_j''(t)dt. \qquad (2.11)$$

Then the roughness is equal to $\xi'K\xi$, so we choose the coefficient vector ξ to minimize $\xi'K\xi$ subject to the constraint $B\xi = x$. If a triangular basis is used, we could use a roughness penalty based on first derivatives, but the principle is the same.

One specific feature of the general approach we have described is that it does not matter if the various functional data in the sample are not observed at the same evaluation points—the procedure will refer all the different functional data to the same basis, regardless of the evaluation points at which each has been observed.

2.5.3 Smoothing the sample mean function

Now we move on to the calculation of the smoothed overall mean and to smoothed principal components analysis. In all cases, it is assumed that we have a set of functional data $Y_1(t), Y_2(t), \ldots, Y_n(t)$ expanded in terms

---

[1] This discussion is subject to the technical condition that B is of full rank. If, exceptionally, this is not so, then a roughness penalty approach can still be used to distinguish between different basis representations that fit the data equally well.

of a basis $\delta_1(t), \ldots, \delta_m(t)$. Thus there is an $n \times m$ matrix $A = (a_{ij})$ of coefficients such that

$$Y_i(t) = \sum_{j=1}^{m} a_{ij}\delta_j(t).$$

If we let $\bar{a}_j = n^{-1}\sum_i a_{ij}$, then we have

$$\bar{Y}(t) = \sum_{j=1}^{m} \bar{a}_j\delta_j(t).$$

Because the basis functions $\delta_j(t)$ may not be sufficiently smooth to allow the appropriate roughness penalty to be defined, we may wish to use a different basis $\beta_k(t)$ of size M when expanding the estimated mean curve. Given an M-vector γ of coefficients, consider the function g with these basis function coefficients in the new basis:

$$g(t) = \sum_{j=1}^{m} \gamma_j\beta_j(t).$$

Define the matrices J and L by

$$J_{ij} = \int \beta_i(t)\beta_j(t)dt \quad \text{and} \quad L_{ij} = \int \beta_i(t)\delta_j(t)dt$$

and the matrix K by (2.11) above.

From these definitions it follows that

$$\int \{g(t) - \bar{Y}(t)\}^2 dt + \lambda \int g''(t)^2 dt = \int \bar{Y}(t)^2 dt + \gamma'J\gamma + \lambda\gamma'K\gamma - 2\gamma'L\bar{a}.$$

By standard linear algebra, this expression is minimized when γ is the vector of coefficients $\gamma^{(\lambda)}$ given by

$$(J + \lambda K)\gamma^{(\lambda)} = L\bar{a}. \tag{2.12}$$

Solving equation (2.12) to find $\gamma^{(\lambda)}$, we can conclude that

$$m_\lambda(t) = \sum_{j=1}^{m} \gamma_j^{(\lambda)}\beta_j(t).$$

2.5.4   Calculations for smoothed functional PCA

Now consider the smoothed functional principal components analysis as discussed in Section 2.3. Suppose that $\xi(t)$ is a possible principal component weight function, and that the vector f gives the coefficients of the basis expansion of $\xi(t)$ in terms of the $\beta_j(t)$, so that

$$\xi(t) = \sum_{j=1}^{m} f_j\beta_j(t).$$

The vector of principal component scores of the data is then

$$\left(\int \xi(t) Y_i(t) dt \right) = AL'f. \tag{2.13}$$

Let V be the sample variance matrix of the basis coefficients of the functional data, so that

$$V_{jk} = (n-1)^{-1} \sum_{i=1}^{n} (a_{ij} - \bar{a}_j)(a_{ik} - \bar{a}_k).$$

The variance of the principal component scores is then $f'LVL'f$. On the other hand, the constraint (2.6) on the size and roughness of $\xi(t)$ is given by

$$\int \xi(t)^2 dt + \alpha \int \xi''(t)^2 dt = f'(J + \alpha K)f = 1. \tag{2.14}$$

To find the leading smoothed principal component, we need to maximize the quadratic form $f'LVL'f$ subject to the constraint (2.14). There are several ways of doing this, but the following approach works well.

Step 1 Use the Choleski decomposition to find a matrix U such that $J + \alpha K = U'U$.

Step 2 Write $g = Uf$ so that $f'(J + \alpha K)f = g'g$. Define $g^{(1)}$ to be the leading eigenvector of the matrix $(U^{-1})'LVL'U^{-1}$. Normalize $g^{(1)}$ to have length 1, so that $g^{(1)}$ maximizes $(U^{-1}g)'LVL'U^{-1}g$ subject to the constraint $g'g = 1$. Set $f^{(1)} = U^{-1}g^{(1)}$. Then $f^{(1)}$ is the basis coefficient vector of the leading smoothed principal component weight function.

Step 3 More generally, let $g^{(j)}$ be the jth normalized eigenvector of $(U^{-1})'LVL'U^{-1}$. Then $U^{-1}g^{(j)}$ is the basis coefficient vector of the jth smoothed principal component weight function.

2.6   Cross-validation for estimating the mean

In classical univariate statistics, the mean of a distribution is the least squares predictor of observations from the distribution, in the sense that if μ is the population mean, and X is a random observation from the distribution, then $E\{(X - \mu)^2\} < E\{(X - a)^2\}$ for any other number a. So one way of evaluating an estimate of μ is to take a number of new observations from the distribution, and see how well they are predicted by the value yielded by our estimate. In the one-dimensional case this may not be a very important issue, but in the functional case, we can use this insight to guide our choice of smoothing parameter.

In an ideal world, we would measure the efficacy of prediction by comparing the estimated mean curve to new functional observations. However, it would take 25 years or more to collect new data! (And, even if we were prepared to wait, the social context would have changed in such a way as to make it impossible to assume the new data came from the same distribution as the original data.) Therefore we have to manufacture the "new observation" situation from our existing data.

The way we do this is to leave each function out in turn from the estimation of the mean. The function left out plays the role of "new data." To be precise, let $m_\lambda^{-i}(t)$ be the smoothed sample mean calculated with smoothing parameter λ from all the data except $Y_i(t)$. To see how well m_λ^{-i} predicts Y_i, we calculate

$$\int \{m_\lambda^{-i}(t) - Y_i(t)\}^2 dt.$$

To avoid edge effects, the integral is taken over a slightly smaller range than that of the data; we integrate over $12 \leq t \leq 34$, but in this case the results are not much affected by this restriction. We now cycle through the whole functional data set and add these integrals together to produce a single measure of the efficacy of the smoothing parameter λ. This quantity is called the *cross-validation score* $CV(\lambda)$; in our case

$$CV(\lambda) = \sum_{i=1}^{413} \int_{12}^{34} \{m_\lambda^{-i}(t) - Y_i(t)\}^2 dt.$$

The smaller the value of $CV(\lambda)$, the better the performance of λ as measured by the cross-validation method.

A plot of the cross-validation score for the criminology data is shown in Figure 2.16. The smoothing parameter value selected by minimizing this score is $\lambda = 2 \times 10^{-7}$. As noted in Figure 2.6, the use of this smoothing parameter yields an estimated mean with some remaining fluctuations that are presumably spurious, and in our context it is appropriate to adjust the smoothing parameter upward a little. In general, it is advisable to use automatic methods such as cross-validation as a guide rather than as a rigid rule.

Before leaving the subject of cross-validation, it is worth pointing out the relation between the cross-validation method we have described here and the standard cross-validation method used in nonparametric regression. In nonparametric regression, we are interested in estimating a curve from a sample (t_i, X_i) of numerical observations X_i taken at time points t_i, and a cross-validation score for a particular smoothing procedure can be found by omitting the X_i one at a time. In the functional case, however, we omit the functional data one at a time, and so the various terms in the cross-validation score relate to the way that a whole function $Y_i(t)$ is predicted from the other functions in the data set.

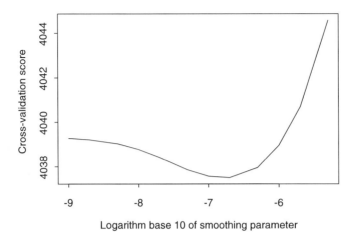

Figure 2.16. Cross-validation score for the estimation of the mean of the criminology data. The smoothing parameter is plotted on a logarithmic scale, and the minimum value is attained at $\lambda = 2 \times 10^{-7}$.

2.7 Notes and bibliography

Glueck and Glueck (1950) describe in detail the way in which the original sample of 500 delinquent boys was constructed and the initial part of the data collection, a process which they continued throughout their careers. A fascinating account of the original collection and processing of the life course data, and the way they were rediscovered, reconstructed, and reinforced is given by Sampson and Laub (1993). Sampson and Laub also describe the methodological controversies within the criminological research community which underlie the interest in the longitudinal analysis of these data.

A general discussion of roughness penalty methods is given in Ramsay and Silverman (1997, Chapter 4), and for a fuller treatment including bibliography the reader is referred to Green and Silverman (1994). The idea of smoothing using roughness penalties has a very long history, going back in some form to the nineteenth century, and certainly to Whittaker (1923). An important early reference to the use of cross-validation to guide the choice of smoothing parameter is Craven and Wahba (1979). In the functional context, the idea of leaving out whole data curves is discussed by Rice and Silverman (1991). The smoothing method for functional principal components analysis described in Section 2.3 is due to Silverman (1996). See also Ramsay and Silverman (1997, Chapter 7).

3
The Nondurable Goods Index

3.1 Introduction

Governments and other institutions use a host of statistical summaries
to track aspects of society across time and space. These range from simple
counts of events such as deaths from lung cancer to sophisticated summaries
of complex processes. For instance, inflation is monitored by the cost of
completing a shopping list carefully designed to reflect the purchases that
most citizens would find essential. To give another example, indices such
as the Dow Jones summarize stock market performance.

The index of nondurable goods manufacturing for the United States,
plotted in Figure 3.1, is a monthly indicator reflecting the producton of
goods that wear out within two years, such as food, tobacco, clothing,
paper products, fuels, and utilities. Because such items are, in normal times,
repeatedly purchased, the index reflects the economy of everyday life. When
times are good, people exhibit strong and stable spending patterns, but
shocks such as the collapse of the stock market in 1929 and the onset of
World War II (1939 in Europe and 1941 in the United States) produce both
short-lived transitory effects, and longer-lasting readjustments of lifestyles.
Technical innovations such as the development of the personal computer
in the early 1980s affect both consumer habits and the production process
itself. You can access these data from the Web site for this chapter.

In this and most economic indicators, there is a multilayered structure.
There are overall trends that span a century or more, and we see in Figure
3.1 that there is a broad tendency for exponential or geometric increase.

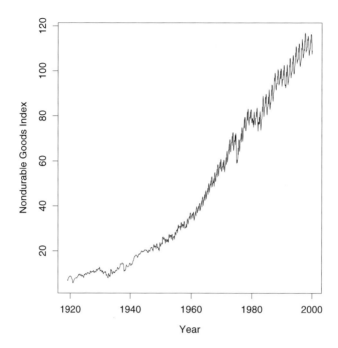

Figure 3.1. Monthly nondurable goods manufacturing for the United States.

Long-term changes last decades, medium-term effects such as recessions last a number of years, and short-term shocks such as the beginning and end of wars are over in a year or two.

We see by the ripples in Figure 3.1 that there is an important seasonal variation in the index. The index includes items often given as gifts, so there is a surge in the index in the last part of each year, followed by a low period in January and February. The beginning of the school year requires new clothes, and we expect to see another surge in the preceding months. On the supply side, though, we need people in the manufacturing process, and vacation periods such as the summer holidays will necessarily have an impact on factory activities.

This seasonal variation is also affected by changes in the economy at various time scales, and so we also want to study how the within-year variation evolves. Perhaps the evolution of seasonal variation can tell us something interesting about how the economy evolves in normal times, and how it reacts to times of crisis and structural change. How did the outbreak of World War II change the seasonal pattern? What about the moving off-shore of a great deal of manufacturing in recent decades? But Figure 3.1 covers too long a time span to reveal much, and we will need to consider some new ways of plotting the seasonal trend.

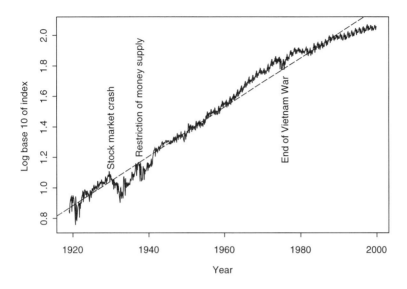

Figure 3.2. The monthly nondurable goods production shown in Figure 3.1 plotted on a logarithmic scale. The dotted straight line is estimated by least squares regression, and has a slope of 0.016, corresponding to a 1.6% increase in the index per year.

3.2 Transformation and smoothing

Like most economic indicators, the nondurable goods index tends to exhibit exponential increase, corresponding to percentage increases over fixed time periods. Moreover, the index tends to increase in size and volatility at the same time, so that the large relative effects surrounding the Second World War seem to be small relative to the large changes in the 1970s and 1980s, and seasonal variation in recent years dwarfs that in early years.

We prefer, therefore, to study the logarithm of this index, displayed in Figure 3.2. The log index has a linear trend with a slope of 0.016, corresponding to an annual rate of increase of 1.6%, and the sizes of the seasonal cycles are also more comparable across time. We now see that the changes in the Great Depression and the war periods are now much more substantial and abrupt than those in recent times. The growth rate is especially high from 1960 to 1975, when the baby boom was in the years of peak consumption; but in subsequent years seems to be substantially lower, perhaps because middle-aged "boomers" consume less, or possibly because the nature of the index itself has changed.

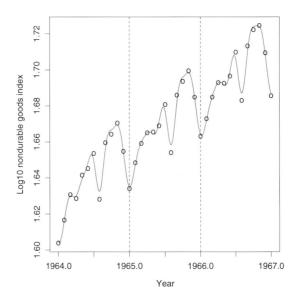

Figure 3.3. The log nondurable goods index for 1964 to 1967, a period of comparative stability. The solid line is a fit to the data using a polynomial smoothing spline. The circles indicate the value of the log index at the first of the month.

A closer look at a comparatively stable period, 1964 to 1967 shown in Figure 3.3, suggests that the index varies fairly smoothly and regularly within each year. The solid line is a smooth of these data using a method described in Section 3.6. We now see that the variation within this year is more complex than Figure 3.2 can possibly reveal. This curve oscillates three times during the year, with the size of the oscillation being smallest in spring, larger in the summer, and largest in the autumn. In fact each year shows smooth variation with a similar amount of detail, and we now consider how we can explore these within-year patterns.

3.3   Phase-plane plots

The rate of change of the index at any point is rather more interesting than its actual size. For example, the increase of 1.6% per year over the twentieth century gives us a reference value or benchmark for the average change of 2.0% from 1963 to 1972 or the smaller 0.8% increase following 1990. The crash of 1929, after all, mattered, not because the index was around 15 at that point, but because it was a change so abrupt that everybody noticed that something had happened.

If, then, it is change that matters, it follows that we need to study whatever alters velocity or the first derivative of the curve. The second derivative of the curve is its acceleration, and is instantaneous curvature in the index. When the index is curving upward, the velocity is increasing. Note the strong positive curvature in the index at the beginning of August, for example.

The smoothing method used to compute the curve in Figure 3.3 was designed to give a good impression of the velocity and acceleration of the log nondurable goods index. The capacity to generate high quality estimates of derivatives as well as curve values is a comparatively recent technical development in statistics and applied mathematics, and more details are provided in Section 3.6.

Now that we have derivatives at our disposal, we can learn new things by studying how derivatives relate to each other. Our tool is the *phase-plane plot*, a plot of acceleration against velocity. To see how this might be useful, consider the phase-plane plot of the function $\sin(2\pi t)$, shown in Figure 3.4. This simple function describes a basic *harmonic process*, such as the vertical position of the end of a suspended spring bouncing with a period of one time unit and starting at position zero at time $t = 0$.

The spring oscillates because energy is exchanged between two states: *potential* and *kinetic*. At times $1, 3, \ldots$ the spring is at one or the other end of its trajectory, and the restorative force due to its stretching has brought it to a standstill. At that point, its potential energy is maximized, and so is the force, which is acting either upward (positively) or downward. Since force is proportional to acceleration, the second derivative of the spring position, $-(2\pi)^2 \sin(2\pi t)$, is also at its highest absolute value, in this case about ± 40. On the other hand, when the spring is passing through the position 0, its velocity, $2\pi \cos(2\pi t)$, is at its greatest, about ± 8, but its acceleration is zero. Since kinetic energy is proportional to the square of velocity, this is the point of highest kinetic energy. The phase-plane plot shows this energy exchange nicely, with potential energy being maximized at the extremes of Y and kinetic energy at the extremes of X.

Now harmonic processes and energy exchange are found in many situations besides mechanics. In economics, potential energy corresponds to available capital, human resources, raw material, and other resources that are at hand to bring about some economic activity, in this case the manufacture of nondurable goods. Kinetic energy corresponds to the manufacturing process in full swing, when these resources are moving along the assembly line, and the goods are being shipped out the factory door.

The process moves from strong kinetic to strong potential energy when the rate of change in production goes to zero. We see this, for example, after a period of rapid increase in production when labor supply and raw material stocks become depleted, and consequently potential energy is actually in a negative state. Or it happens when management winds down produc-

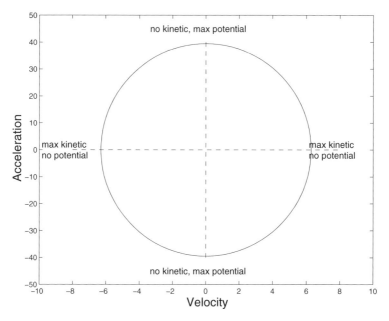

Figure 3.4. A phase-plane plot of the simple harmonic function $\sin(2\pi t)$. Kinetic energy is maximized when acceleration is 0, and potential energy is maximized when velocity is 0.

tion because targets have been achieved, so that personnel and material resources are piling up and waiting to be used anew.

After a period of intense production, or at certain periods of crisis that we examine shortly, we may see that both potential and kinetic energy are low. This corresponds to a period when the phase-plane curve is closer to zero than is otherwise the case.

To summarize, here's what we are looking for:

- a substantial cycle;

- the size of the radius: the larger it is, the more energy transfer there is in the event;

- the horizontal location of the center: if it is to the right, there is net positive velocity, and if to the left, there is net negative velocity;

- the vertical location of the center: if it is above zero, there is net velocity increase; if below zero, there is velocity decrease; and

- changes in the shapes of the cycles from year to year.

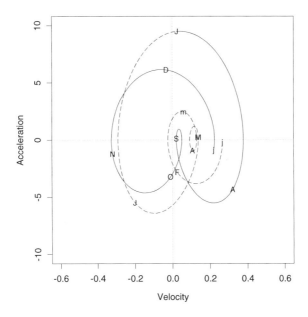

Figure 3.5. A phase-plane plot of the first derivative or velocity and the second derivative or acceleration of the smoothed log nondurable goods index for 1964. Letters indicate midmonths, with lowercase letters used for January and March. For clarity, the first half of the year is plotted as a dashed line, and the second half as a solid line.

3.4   The nondurable goods cycles

We use the phase-plane plot, therefore, to study the energy transfer within the economic system. We can examine the cycle within individual years, and also see more clearly how the structure of the transfer has changed throughout the twentieth century. Figure 3.5 phase-plane plots the year 1964, a year in a relatively stable period for the index. To read the plot, find the lower-case "j" in the middle right of the plot, and move around the diagram clockwise, noting the letters indicating the months as you go. You will see that there are two large cycles surrounding zero, plus some small cycles that are much closer to the origin.

The largest cycle begins in mid-May (M), with positive velocity but near zero acceleration. Production is increasing linearly or steadily at this point. The cycle moves clockwise through June (first J) and passes the horizontal zero acceleration line at the end of the month, when production is now decreasing linearly. By mid-July (second J) kinetic energy or velocity is near zero because vacation season is in full swing. But potential energy or acceleration is high, and production returns to the positive kinetic/zero potential phase in early August (A), and finally concludes with a cusp at summer's end (S). At this point the process looks like it has run out of both potential and kinetic energy.

The cusp, near where both derivatives are zero, corresponds to the start of school in September, and to the beginning of the next big production cycle passing through the autumn months of October through November. Again this large cycle terminates in a small cycle with little potential and kinetic energy. This takes up the months of February and March (F and m). The tiny subcycle during April and May seems to be due to the spring holidays, since the summer and fall cycles, as well as the cusp, don't change much over the next two years, but the spring cycle cusp moves around, reflecting the variability in the timings of Easter and Passover.

To summarize, the production year in the 1960s has two large cycles swinging widely around zero, each terminating in a small cusplike cycle. This suggests that each large cycle is like a balloon that runs out of air, the first at the beginning of school, and the second at the end of winter. At the end of each cycle, it may be that new resources must be marshaled before the next production cycle can begin.

With this basic pattern characterizing the phase-plane plot for a stable year, it can be revealing to examine years in which important events took place. Figure 3.6 shows what happened in 1929 to 1931. Year 1929 has the same features as we saw above for 1964, but we see a bulge to the left in the late autumn, when the stock market crashed. By November of that year production was in a state of freefall. We pick up the story in the middle cycle for 1930, and see that, after a small spring and larger summer cycle, the autumn cycle loses much of its potential energy, and this is even more evident in 1931. Probably this is attributable to the collapse of consumer demand in the holiday period as people restrict spending to the essentials.

Figure 3.7 pictures the events leading to World War II. The first part of 1937 shows only small amounts of energy as the Depression continues. But the cycle is dramatically altered in the fall by the sudden decrease in the money supply imposed by the Treasury Board when it feared that the economy might be overheated and headed for another crash. You can see in Figure 3.2 that this precipitous event is comparable in size to the stock market crash of 1929, but even more sudden. The spring and fall cycles were all but wiped out in 1938.

The bottom plot in Figure 3.7 shows the reduced seasonal variability during the war years, and this is also clearly visible in Figure 3.2. In times of war people don't take holidays, make do with what they have, and spend less at Christmas. Moreover, war production did not exhibit much seasonal variation since the demand for nondurable goods, like the war itself, was steady through the year.

Another three years in which important changes occur are 1974 to 1976, plotted in Figure 3.8. The Vietnam War was concluded in this period, and

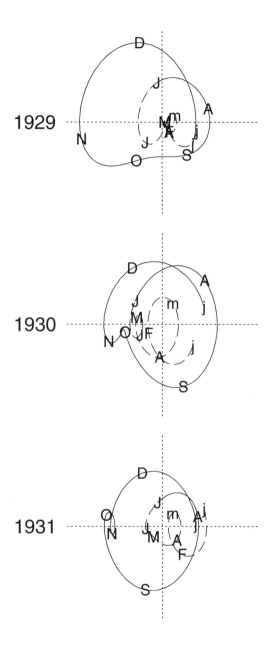

Figure 3.6. Phase-plane plots for the years 1929 to 1931, during the onset of the Great Depression. The horizontal and vertical scale is the same as in Figure 3.5.

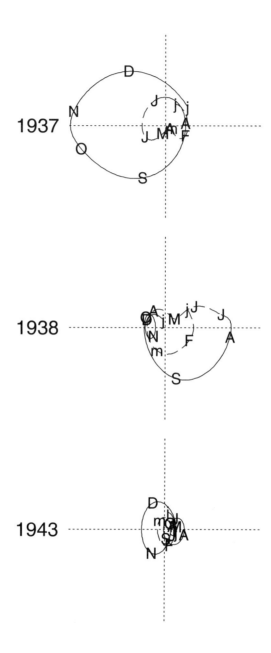

Figure 3.7. Phase-plane plots for two years preceding the Second World War and a typical war year.

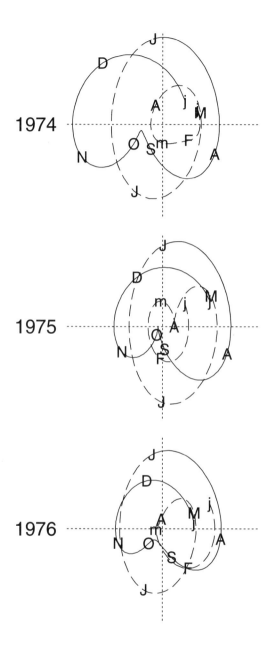

Figure 3.8. Phase-plane plots for 1974 to 1976, when the production cycles are changing rapidly.

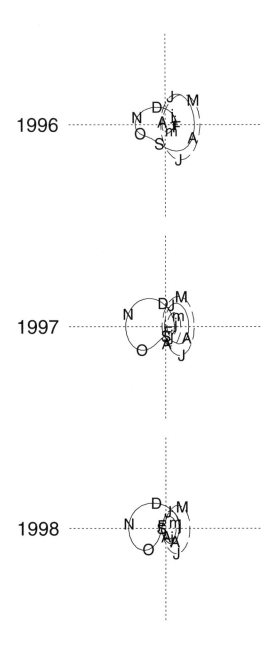

Figure 3.9. Phase-plane plots for 1996 to 1998, showing the greatly reduced variability of current production cycles.

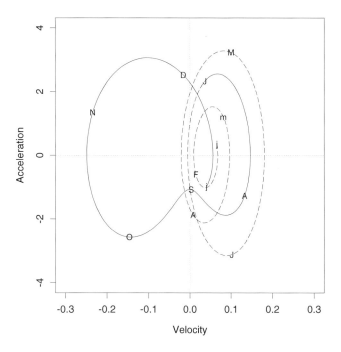

Figure 3.10. The phase-plane plot for 1997 on a larger scale, showing the structural changes in current production cycles.

the OPEC oil crisis also contributed to a change in economic patterns. One consequence was the decrease in the size of the fall loop. What we cannot see in this small time window, though, is that fundamental changes initiated in the mid-1970s persist to the present day.

What is happening now? Figure 3.9 shows that the production cycles are now much smaller than they once were. We still see fairly large seasonal oscillations, but they are now much smoother, and hence show less variation in velocity and acceleration. Also, if we look at Figure 3.10 showing the 1997 cycles on a larger scale, we see that there are now four cycles rather than three, and that the final winter cycle has a strongly negative net velocity. Are this loss of dynamism and these structural changes due to the fact that production is no longer so dependent on manpower? Or, perhaps, that it is more tightly controlled by information technology? On the other hand, it may be simply that far more nondurable goods are now manufactured outside the United States.

A further clue to recent changes is that in the early 1990s, personal computers and other electronic goods were classified as durable. Consequently, one sees in the comparable index for durable goods a strong increase in its typical slope at that point. Although it is true that electronic goods usually last more than two years, the pace of technological development in this sector has meant that, effectively, consumers have tended to discard these items because they are obsolete. This loss of electronic goods in the nondurable goods index has surely diminished its energy.

3.5   What have we seen?

Phase-plane plotting is revealing because it focuses our attention on the *dynamics* of the seasonal component of variation in the goods index. We plot velocity on the horizontal axis, representing the rate of change of the process; and plot acceleration on the vertical axis, indicating the input or withdrawal of whatever resources or forces produce this change. Because seasonal components tend to exhibit oscillatory or harmonic behavior, we can interpret what we see as a transition between two types of energy: kinetic associated with velocity, and potential associated with acceleration. Harmonic behavior, in which the system moves between these two states, shows up as a loop surrounding the origin. The bigger the radius of the loop, the more energy the system has, and the smaller or closer it is to zero, the less the energy.

We saw that the typical year shows three such loops, associated with the spring, summer, and fall. The summer loop typically has the largest associated energy. But the fall loop seems to be most affected by shocks such as the stock market crash of 1929, the shutting down of the money supply in 1937, and the end of the Vietnam War in 1974. This is probably due to the fact that the fall production loop is associated with buying for the Christmas holidays, and therefore is something consumers can turn on and off according to whether times are good or tough, respectively.

We also saw the seasonal dynamics reflecting longer-term changes. There is much less energy in the system now than in the 1960s, as reflected in the smallness of loops in recent times.

The dynamics of a process typically show more variation than the statics or position of the process, and we could see things happening in the phase-plane plots that would be hard to spot in the plot of the process itself, such as in Figure 3.2.

This focus on dynamics leads to the question of whether we can model these dynamic features directly, rather than putting all of our statistical energy into reproducing the curve itself. This leads us naturally to the idea of using a *differential equation* to describe the process, a type of modeling that will allow us to model the dynamic behavior seen in the phase-plane plot as well as the curve itself. We use differential equations in models in Chapters 11 and 12.

3.6   Smoothing data for phase-plane plots

3.6.1   Fourth derivative roughness penalties

We can imagine that the economic forces generating the log index values are reasonably smooth. In practice, this means that a curve giving a satisfactory picture of these processes has a certain number of derivatives. For phase-plane plotting, in particular, we need to use two derivatives in addition to the curve values themselves. We estimate these derivatives by smoothing the data, using a method that will give useful estimates of velocity and acceleration as well as of the underlying curve itself.

Therefore we choose to fit a smooth curve $h(t)$ to log index values $y_i, i = 1, \ldots, 973$, by using the following criterion

$$\text{PENSSE}_\lambda(h) = \sum_{i=1}^{973} [y_i - h(t_i)]^2 + \lambda \int_{1919}^{2000} [h^{(iv)}(t)]^2 \, dt. \qquad (3.1)$$

The criterion has two terms. The first assesses the fidelity of the curve to the observed data in the sense of the sum of squared errors.

But fitting the data is not our only concern, and the second term, the penalty term, measures the extent to which the fitting function $h(t)$ is smooth. The notation $h^{(iv)}(t)$ in (3.1) means the fourth derivative of h evaluated at time t. The penalty term captures the overall size of this fourth derivative by integrating its square over the interval of interest. Why the fourth derivative? Because it is sensitive to the curvature of the second derivative, or acceleration. Recall that curvature is indicated by the second derivative, so the curvature of the acceleration function is its second derivative, or the fourth derivative of the actual curve $h(t)$.

We cannot have smoothness and a nearly perfect fit to the data at the same time, especially when we have this many observations. The smoothing parameter λ controls the relative emphasis on fitting the data and smoothness. As λ increases, smoothness is accentuated more and more, until finally the integrated square of $h^{(iv)}(t)$ will be driven to zero. Only polynomials of degree three or fewer have zero fourth derivatives, and clearly a function this simple would not fit these data at all well. On the other hand, as λ goes to zero, smoothness matters less and less, and hence fitting the data more and more. Finally we will arrive at a function that fits the data exactly. Unfortunately, it will not be at all smooth, and its second derivative will be too wildly varying to be at all useful. The challenge, then, is to find a value for λ that works for us.

3.6.2   Choosing the smoothing parameter

We discussed this problem in Chapter 2. There a data-driven technique, cross-validation, was described that could be used to guide this choice. However, we were not shy to say that our final choice depended on inspection of the results, and that we used a value rather different than that suggested by this purely data-driven method. We now continue to discuss concerns that might govern the amount of smoothness in a curve that smooths data.

Our goal in this chapter was to use phase-plane plots to reveal something about seasonal trend, and how it evolves over time. Of course the technique is not going to be helpful if the curve misses obviously important features in the data. Our first move, therefore, was to carefully study how well the curve tracks the data by using close-up plots such as Figure 3.3. We actually plotted the data and the fit separately for each of the 51 years of interest, and noted where the curve seemed to miss the data repeatedly. We observed, for example, that the curve was too smooth if it underestimated peak values such as that of June year after year, or if it consistently overestimated low values such as July. We also learned a lot by looking at the residuals from the fit, computed by subtracting the fitted from the actual value. If there was some trend running over several months, this was a sign that we had oversmoothed the data. At this stage, one may say, it is rather easier to detect oversmoothing than undersmoothing. These investigations gave us a fairly firm idea of an upper limit on λ, but less intuition about a lower limit.

Next we looked at what we wanted to work with, namely the phase-plane plot. Here smoothness matters a great deal. We wanted to see important and consistent patterns, and too much wiggliness in the plot makes this difficult. In general, high derivatives are rather more unstable than lower ones, so at this point it was primarily smoothness in acceleration that mattered; if acceleration was smooth, so was velocity. So we started with a smallish value of λ, and moved it upward bit by bit until the phase-plane plot seemed stable from year to year over periods when it should be, such as the 1960s, and, of course, to the point where we could make sense out of the structure of the plot. This process gave us a desirable lower limit on λ.

We have to admit that this lower limit is often larger than the upper limit identified by looking at the data fit. However, at this point some fit just has to be sacrificed in order to see what we are looking for in the data—hence the systematic misfitting of the July log index in Figure 3.3. Perhaps we will return to the data someday to have a look at what we missed this time, but for the moment we are satisfied with what we learned. Our final choice for λ was $10^{-9.5}$.

In summary, our philosophy, and, we believe, the perspective of most practitioners of smoothing, is that choosing a level of smoothing is a matter of balancing off fitting the data against getting a stable and interpretable estimate of what interests us. We see the choice of λ as very much driven by the needs of the investigator, and are content to see other analyses of the same data employ a different value.

4
Bone Shapes from a Paleopathology Study

4.1   Archaeology and arthritis

Archaeologists have conducted a major excavation at St. Peter's Church, Barton-upon-Humber, in the north of England. They have exhumed the skeletons of about 2000 adults dating mainly from between 1000 and 1500 C.E. A particular way in which the bones have been studied is for *paleopathology*—the use of old remains to give us information about diseases that people suffered from in the past. Many diseases leave traces on the bones, and special attention was given to osteoarthritis of the knee, both because it is and was a common and painful disease, and because the skeletal remains give us easy access to parts of the knee joint not easily seen on X-rays.

The paleopathologists attempted to identify every person in the sample with definite signs of osteoarthritis of the knee, as evidenced by *eburnation*—polished bone surface caused by complete cartilage loss. Initially, 23 people were found with eburnation on at least one femur. For each such person, controls matched approximately by age, sex, and period of burial were found from among those with no evidence of osteoarthritis at any joint. Once the joints with postmortem damage had been eliminated, this left 16 eburnated femora and 52 controls for analysis.

Several aspects of the biomechanics of the knee have been studied in relation to osteoarthritis. These include obesity, injury, and lower limb malalignment, but the shape of the joint itself has not been very much considered. It has been hypothesized that osteoarthritis can affect bone

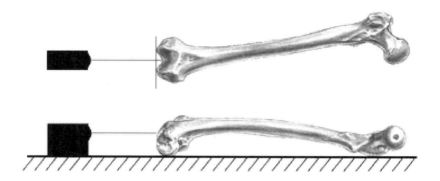

Figure 4.1. Setup showing how the image is captured. A camera captured a digital image of each bone. From Shepstone et al. (1999).

shape, or conversely that certain joint shapes may affect the biomechanics of the joint and hence increase the risk of osteoarthritis. It is against this background that a study of the shapes of the bones was carried out.

4.2   Data capture

As is typical, the investigation had to be carried out rapidly and with a low budget, and so it was not possible to study the three-dimensional structure directly. However, very interesting conclusions can be drawn from simpler two-dimensional images of the joint shape. The first step was to capture the data themselves. Each bone was photographed end-on, as in Figure 4.1, to yield an image as shown in Figure 1.5.

The easiest way of identifying the shape of the joint was to "mark up" each image on the screen by direct reference to the actual bone. The result was a pixel image, with certain pixels specified as being within the outline of the joint. All left femora were reflected to produce "right" images, in order to give every bone a consistent orientation. A typical image is shown in Figure 4.2. The knee end forms an inverted U-shape. The two arms of the inverted U-shape formed by the knee are called *condyles*, and the space between them is the *intercondylar notch*. The smaller indentation at the top of the image is called the *patellar groove*.

For our analysis, we have 68 outlines, of which some are known to correspond to arthritic joints. We regard each outline as a single data object, and consider ways of studying the variability in shape between the bones, and of relating this variability to the presence or absence of arthritis. The first step in studying the shapes is to parameterize the images in an appropriate way. One way of doing this is by defining landmarks; these give a natural way of representing a shape by a fairly low-dimensional array of

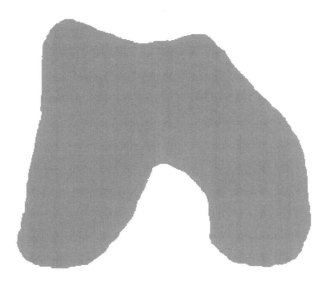

Figure 4.2. Bitmap image after drawing round the outline in Figure 1.5 on the screen and reversing to yield standard orientation.

numbers. In Chapter 8 we return to these data and consider a different approach concentrating on the intercondylar notch alone.

4.3 How are the shapes parameterized?

The principle of using landmarks is to locate a fairly small collection of points from which the shape itself can be reasonably reconstructed. The process used for the bone shapes is best described by reference to Figure 4.3. Initially, the landmarks numbered 1, 2, 5, 7, 9, and 12 were located 'by hand' (in fact by mouse) on the image. These correspond to lowest and highest points on the relevant part of the outline, but because of the strange shapes of some of the specimens, are easier located manually than algorithmically. Then landmarks 3, 6, 8, and 11 were defined as the extreme points within the image of the perpendicular bisector of the lines 2–5, 5–7, 7–9 and 9–12 respectively. This process was repeated on the lines 3–5 and 9–11 to give landmarks 4 and 10. For the remainder of the analysis, we discarded the bone pixel images and worked with the landmarks.

Any bone's shape can be reasonably well approximated by putting a smooth curve through the coordinates of the 12 landmarks. Although the calculations we carry out are in terms of the 24 coordinates of the landmarks, conceptually we are considering the shapes as the data of interest,

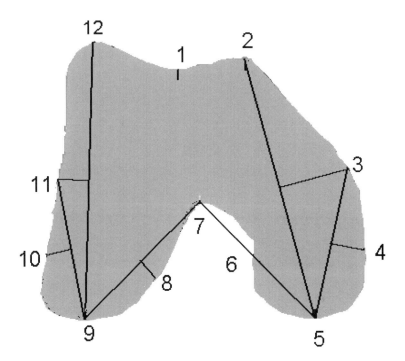

Figure 4.3. Demonstration of the process of identifying and constructing land-marks. Landmarks 1, 2, 5, 7, 9, and 12 are located manually, and the others are then found automatically, as the extreme points within the image of the perpendicular bisector of the lines shown. From Shepstone et al. (1999).

and the results in terms of the curves themselves. To each set of landmark positions there corresponds a periodic curve, and the coordinates of the landmarks are the way that the curves are represented internally to our calculations.

To be precise, the interpolation is carried out by fitting periodic cubic spline interpolants to the landmark x and y values separately, to give functions $x(t)$ and $y(t)$ for t in $[0, 1]$. A cubic spline is a curve made of pieces of cubic polynomials, joined together smoothly at the data points, and the fitting was done using the S-PLUS routine `spline`. The landmark positions gave the values of x and y at the points $i/12$ for $i = 1, 2, \ldots, 12$. As t varies, the point $(x(t), y(t))$ then traces out the curve. The same technique is used whenever we wish to recover a curve from its landmark positions. In mathematical terms, continuing the ideas discussed in Section 2.5, we have implicitly constructed a basis for the representation of these shapes.

4.4   A functional principal components analysis

4.4.1   Procrustes rotation and PCA calculation

Because the size and orientation of the bones is of no particular interest, we eliminate size and orientation variability by a process known as *Procrustes transformation*. In Greek mythology, Procrustes was a robber who captured passing travelers and made them fit his bed, either by stretching their limbs or by chopping them off. Fortunately the analysis of data is less traumatic, but the idea is still to adjust the data so they fit together as closely as possible. First each configuration is centered at its mean, in order to eliminate any translation effects. Then the configurations are all rotated and scaled to minimize the sum of squares between the configurations. For software details, see the Web page associated with this chapter.

Let $\mu_1, \mu_2, \ldots, \mu_{12}$ be the mean positions of the 12 landmarks, after transformation. Let μ be the interpolating curve between these positions, constructed in the way described in Section 4.3. Then μ is considered as the mean bone shape.

Each individual shape yields a vector of 24 coordinates, the x and y coordinates of the 12 landmarks. (Because of the Procrustes fitting, there are some dependences between these coordinates, but that does not affect the subsequent work.) We perform a functional principal components analysis of the 68 curves by using standard principal components analysis on the 68 24-vectors of landmark coordinates. Before examining the results, it is worth reviewing the way in which this functional principal components analysis can be interpreted.

4.4.2   Visualizing the components of shape variability

Concentrate first on the leading component. For this component, standard PCA provides a 24-vector of principal component loadings, which can be expressed as twelve 2-vectors $\mathbf{z}_1, \mathbf{z}_2, \ldots, \mathbf{z}_{12}$. As we saw in Section 2.3, a good way of visualizing the relevant variation is to plot curves corresponding to the mean plus and minus a multiple of the effect of variation in this component direction. Indeed, in the shape context it is hardly meaningful to consider the principal component weights aside from their effect on a particular shape such as the mean. In the present example, three standard deviations of the principal component give a suitable multiple; more generally the choice may have to be adjusted subjectively.

Let s be the sample standard deviation of the principal component. We then find two curves, plotted in Figure 4.4. The solid curve is the interpolant to the landmarks $\mu_1 + 3s\mathbf{z}_1, \mu_2 + 3s\mathbf{z}_2, \ldots, \mu_{12} + 3s\mathbf{z}_{12}$. The first principal component of this curve will be $3s$, and it will exemplify the kind of curve that has a positive value of the first principal component. The dashed curve is the interpolant to $\mu_1 - 3s\mathbf{z}_1, \mu_2 - 3s\mathbf{z}_2, \ldots, \mu_{12} - 3s\mathbf{z}_{12}$, and will have

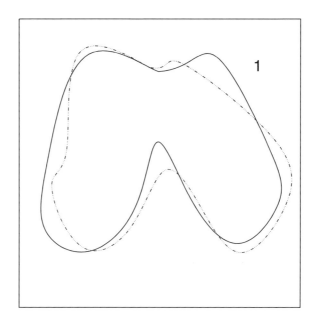

Figure 4.4. The effect of the first principal component of variation. The curves correspond to the mean ± three standard deviations of the component. The solid curve is the effect of adding the component and the dashed curve of subtracting it. This component explains 21% of the variability in the original data.

a negative value of the first principal component. Furthermore, the two curves indicate the variability of the first principal component within the data, because of the choice of a multiple depending on s. In the present case we do not plot the mean shape itself, because the mean can be inferred by eye from the given curves.

It can be seen from Figure 4.4 that if an outline has a positive score on the first principal component, then we can expect it to have a deeper intercondylar notch, and also a more pronounced bulge in the top right part of the image. The converse characteristics would be associated with a negative value of this component.

Similar plots for each of the principal components 2 to 5 are shown in Figure 4.5. The second component will be of particular importance; a positive score is associated with a narrowing of the right-hand condyle (in our diagram) and with a deepening and widening of the intercondylar notch.

How do arthritic bones differ from controls? For each component, a t-test was carried out to compare the eburnated and noneburnated bones. There was no significant difference on components 1, 3, 4, and 5, but the difference on component 2 was highly significant ($t = -3.01$, $p = 0.0037$). On this component, the mean for the eburnated bones was -10.9 and for

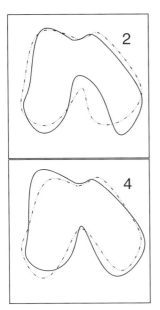
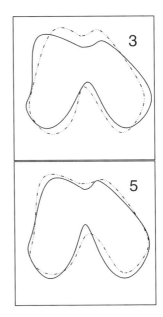

Figure 4.5. The effects of the second to fifth principal components of variation. These explain 18%, 12%, 9%, and 8% of the original variability, respectively. Only on the second component is there a significant difference ($p = 0.0037$) between the eburnated and noneburnated bones. On this component the mean score for the eburnated bones was significantly higher than for the controls.

the controls it was 3.4. This indicates that, on the average, the eburnated bones will tend to have the properties associated with a positive score on component 2.

4.5 Varimax rotation of the principal components

It is well known in classical multivariate analysis that an appropriate rotation of the principal components can, on occasion, give components of variability more informative than the original components themselves. A rotation method constructs new components based on the first k principal components, for some relatively small k. The idea is that k is chosen to include all the components that convey meaningful information, but not those that are just "noise". In the present example, we concentrate on the first five components and set $k = 5$.

The varimax method is often a useful approach. The method chooses components to maximize the variability of the *squared* principal component weights. The resulting modes of variability tend to be concentrated on part of the range of the function in question, so in the present context

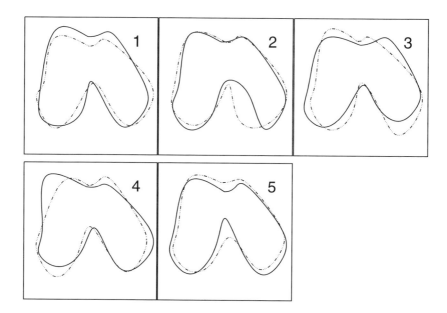

Figure 4.6. The effects of the first five varimax-rotated components for the bone shape data. The percentages of variability explained are, respectively, 14%, 15%, 15%, 11%, and 13%. The arthritic bones had significantly higher scores than the controls on component 2 and significantly lower on component 3.

they express departures from the mean curve over part of the outline shape rather than the whole of it. They are still orthogonal, but the values of the components for the data will no longer necessarily be uncorrelated. Furthermore, the variances of the varimax components will be less spread out than those of ordinary components, and need no longer decrease monotonically. The varimax algorithm is discussed further in Section 4.8.

The modes of variation corresponding to the varimax-rotated components are shown in Figure 4.6. Compared to the original principal components in Figures 4.4 and 4.5, some of the varimax components are more definitely interpretable in terms of the bone shape. Varimax component 2 completely corresponds to a thinner right condyle, in the orientation shown in the figure. Component 5 is concentrated almost entirely on a much narrower join between the condyles. Component 3 is associated with a broader intercondylar notch, but more particularly with a much more symmetric patellar groove than the mean.

The percentages of variances explained by the components are roughly the same for each of the components displayed. As with the raw principal components, the component scores for the two classes of bones were compared. On components 2 and 3 the difference is significant, but not as strongly as previously ($p < 0.025$ in both cases). On component 2 the eburnated bones tend to have negative scores, whereas their scores on component 3 tend to be larger than average. This suggests that the eburnated bones tend to have a thicker right condyle, and a flatter and more symmetric patellar groove.

Is varimax rotation worthwhile? It yields components that have much more direct meaning for the bone shapes themselves. In terms of finding ways in which the two groups of bones differ, it highlights two components rather than concentrating attention on a single component. However, the individual interpretation of each of these two components, especially varimax component 2, is much more physically intuitive than the composite effect represented by original component 2 in Figure 4.4.

4.6   Bone shapes and arthritis: Clinical relationship?

The relationship between the shape of the femur and the incidence of osteoarthritis of the knee has not been studied widely, and so any clinical conclusions have to be tentative. It is possible to analyze the data further, for example, by breaking down the eburnated group according to the position of the eburnation. There is then some suggestion that the location of the eburnation is associated with the third varimax-rotated component score, corresponding to the variation in shape of the patellar groove. On the other hand, the change in shape of the condyles associated with the second varimax component seems only to be associated with presence or absence of eburnation. However, the numbers of bones in each subgroup are not sufficient to draw firm conclusions.

What is the possible link between arthritis and the shape of the bones? On the basis of these data alone, it is not possible to discover to what extent shape variation in the condyle is a cause or an effect of osteoarthritis. Differences in intercondylar notch shape could conceivably affect the functioning of the ligaments in the joint, or increase the likelihood of damage, and lead to an increased risk of knee osteoarthritis. Conversely, arthritis causes a change in biomechanics, which could possibly lead to bone remodeling. An increase in the width of the condyle would help to stabilize an unstable joint or dissipate increased pressure. The data support the concept of a feedback mechanism within which this kind of reshaping of joints is an attempt to slow, or counter, the effects of osteoarthritis.

The association of eburnation with the shape of the patellar groove is more of a puzzle. Postmortem studies have shown a naturally occurring wide variation in patellar groove shape. This could be a potential risk factor, with a wide and shallow groove leading to biomechanical differences that can cause osteoarthritis. However, the potential mechanisms are not yet well understood.

4.7   What have we seen?

Functional data do not have to be a simple function of one variable, but can take many other forms. For the analysis of the bone shape data, the functions of interest were shapes as described by cyclic curves in two dimensions. An interesting topic for future research would be the consideration of the full three-dimensional joint shape; leaving aside statistical considerations, in the present context this would have been impossible because appropriate data-collection equipment was not available.

Landmarks can provide a very good way of representing functional data. We think about our data as functions, but we have to represent them in a finite-dimensional way in order to carry out calculations, and landmarks are one way of getting a finite-dimensional representation. The landmarks may or may not be of direct interest in themselves—in this chapter they were only the means to the end of considering the function as a whole.

Principal components analysis gave us the way of identifying important modes of variability in the data. In some data sets we would study the values of the principal components on individuals, but in this case it was of particular interest to compare two groups, the eburnated and the noneburnated bones. Once the principal component scores had been found, standard statistical techniques could be used to compare the groups.

The varimax procedure improved the interpretability of the components to some extent, and also was useful in subsequent analysis taking into account the position of eburnation. Varimax and other rotation methods are not a panacea, but will often provide a helpful contribution to the analysis of the data.

4.8   Notes and bibliography

Much of the material of this chapter is based on Shepstone, Rogers, Kirwan, and Silverman (1999), although the method of varimax rotation is somewhat different. They give details of data collection and of the arthritis background, with many references to the relevant literature. They also give further discussion of the conclusions drawn in Section 4.6 above. The data collection from the original bones was carried out as part of Lee Shepstone's Ph.D. research (Shepstone, 1998), under the supervision of the other three authors of the paper.

The use of landmarks to characterize curves is discussed in Ramsay and Silverman (1997, Chapter 5). Dryden and Mardia (1998) give a full discussion of landmark-based methods of the analysis of shape data, together with many references to the literature on statistics of shape. For more material and references on functional PCA, see Ramsay and Silverman (1997, Chapter 6). Their Section 6.3.3 gives some discussion of the varimax-rotation procedure. Fuller details of varimax rotation, and also of Procrustes fitting, are given in standard multivariate text books. See, for example, Harman (1976), or Mardia, Kent, and Bibby (1979).

There is a subtle point to be taken into account in the case we have discussed. Each landmark is a 2-vector, and so the principal component weights are themselves 2-vectors. We therefore base the varimax criterion on the variability of the squared lengths of the 2-vectors of principal component weights, rather than directly on the individual weights. Suppose that the loadings of the first five principal component weights are given by two 12×5 matrices $\mathbf{A}^X$ and $\mathbf{A}^Y$, respectively containing the loadings on the x- and y-coordinates of the 12 landmarks. We aim to find a 5×5 rotation matrix $\mathbf{T}$, yielding rotated loadings matrices $\mathbf{B}^X = \mathbf{A}^X\mathbf{T}$ and $\mathbf{B}^Y = \mathbf{A}^Y\mathbf{T}$, to maximize the variance of the quantity

$$\sum_{i=1}^{12}\sum_{k=1}^{5}||b_{ik}||^2,$$

where b_{ik} is the 2-vector $(\mathbf{B}^X_{ik}, \mathbf{B}^Y_{ik})$. See the Web page for this chapter for further details.

5

Modeling Reaction-Time Distributions

5.1 Introduction

Hyperactivity in children has been a hot topic in recent years among educational and psychological researchers, not to mention doctors, nurses, and other health professionals. The technical term, attention deficit (hyperactive) disorder, or ADHD, captures the central issue, the difficulty these children have in focusing their attention on tasks for more than brief periods. This affliction is especially troublesome in school.

In spite of the popularity of the term, hyperactivity is actually difficult to diagnose, and may even be rather rare. Because of the frequency with which certain drugs are prescribed to calm down supposedly hyperactive children, as well as the need to test more carefully the efficacy of these drugs, it is imperative to find clearcut techniques to identify the ADHD syndrome.

One behavioral marker is the time taken to react to a visual stimulus appearing after a warning signal, but with a substantial delay. In a typical experiment, children see a warning on a computer screen that a light is about to appear, and are required to push a key as rapidly as possible when a light actually appears. When there is a delay of 10 seconds or so, ADHD individuals not only take longer to react on the average, presumably because their attention has wandered, but they also show a higher frequency of extremely long reaction times.

Figure 5.1 displays two reaction-time distributions, one for the first child in a sample of 17 ADHD children, and another for the first child in a sam-

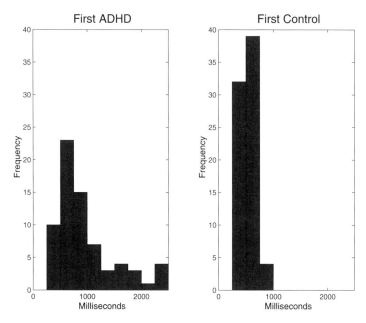

Figure 5.1. Histograms for about 70 reaction times to the onset of a signal after an eight-second delay. The left histogram is for the first of a sample of 17 attention deficit (hyperactive) disorder children, and the right for an age-matched control child.

ple of 16 age-matched control children. Each histogram is computed from about 70 reaction times. The experiment is described in Leth-Steenson, King Elbaz, and Douglas (2000). We see that the ADHD child has many reaction times beyond one second, while the control child never takes that long to respond.

A histogram, such as those in Figure 5.1, gives us only a crude impression of a distribution, and we would prefer to work with the probability density function $p(t)$, describing the reaction-time distributions. This would permit us to calculate the probability of a reaction time between two limits, t_0 and t_1, as

$$\text{Prob}\{t_0 \leq t \leq t_1\} = \int_{t_0}^{t_1} p(t)\, dt \ .$$

But researchers who work with reaction times know that none of the standard textbook distributions capture the features of reaction-time distributions. These characteristics include

- an initial period of at least 120 milliseconds in which no reaction is possible,

- a rapid increase in the number of reaction times after this dead time,

- a strong positive skewness, and

- a very long tail with a severe tendency to outliers.

In these data, for example, we considered reaction times longer than three seconds to be outliers and did not use them, since the large majority of reaction times even for the ADHD children occurred in less time. The shortest reaction time observed was 239 milliseconds.

These distributional features reflect the sequence of neural activities that must precede a reaction, including passage of peripheral excitation to the brain, processing of this information to yield a decision, assembly of the excitation patterns required to generate a response, transmission of these to the neural/muscle interfaces, and delays within muscle tissues before an observable response is possible. All this is compounded by intrusions of attentional lapses, other higher priority events such as a sneeze, and so forth.

We therefore want to explore the implications of ADHD for reaction times without relying on parametric models for the reaction-time distributions. At the same time, we also want to explore the variation in reaction-time distributions from child to child within each group. Our perspective here is that we have two samples of reaction-time distributions, each distribution being identified by around 70 observations. After eliminating reaction times that exceeded three seconds, there were 1111 reaction times for the normal control group, and 1138 for the ADHD group. Our objective is to use functional principal components analysis within each sample to get some picture of the typical modes of variation. But this raises a technical issue: Density functions are by definition positive and integrate to one, but functional principal components analysis is more naturally applied to families of unconstrained functions. It is with this issue in mind that we consider methods of density estimation and modeling that avoid the constraints implicit in the definition of a density function.

5.2   Nonparametric modeling of density functions

A probability density $p(t)$ must satisfy the constraints

- $p(t) > 0$ over some interval $[t_L, t_U]$ of interest, and

- the area under this curve is one; that is,

$$\int_{t_L}^{t_U} p(t)\, dt = 1 .$$

Given any function $W(t)$, we can construct a probability density function $p(t)$ by

$$p(t) = C \exp W(t), \tag{5.1}$$

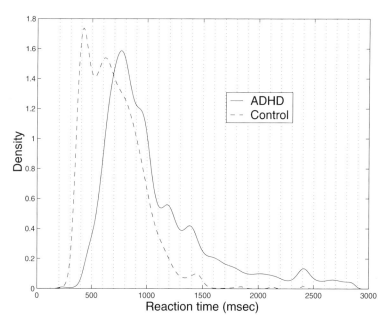

Figure 5.2. The solid curve is the density function for 1143 reaction times observed for the 17 ADHD children, and the dashed curve the density function for 1113 times for the 16 control children. The vertical dotted lines indicate the knot placement in the B-spline basis described in Section 5.6. The smoothing method requires the choice of a smoothing parameter λ, which was set to 10^6. The density values have been multiplied by 1000.

where

$$C = \Big[\int_{t_L}^{t_U} \exp W(x)\, dx \Big]^{-1}.$$

Without any constraints on the function $W(t)$, the conditions for $p(t)$ to be a probability density function will be satisfied automatically. The function $W(t)$ and hence the density $p(t)$ can be estimated by a *penalized maximum likelihood* method, as described in Section 5.6.

Figure 5.2 displays the density functions estimated for the combined data for the two groups. We see that even the fast ADHD times are slower by around 200 milliseconds than fast times for the controls. For example, for the ADHD group, only 8% of the times are faster than 600 msec, compared with the control group which has 40% of the times. We also see that the distributions show some bimodality, and even a hint of trimodality. A distinctive feature of the ADHD times is the large shoulder and long tail on the positive side of the distribution. For example, fewer than 1% of control group times exceed 1600 msec, as compared to 12% of the ADHD times.

The two densities in Figure 5.2, however, ignore individual differences in response times, and in particular, are likely to have more spread than

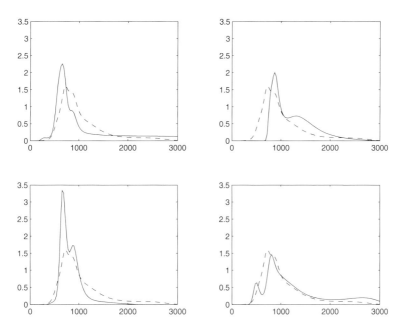

Figure 5.3. Individual reaction-time densities for four of the ADHD children (solid curve) along with the reaction-time density estimated for the entire group (dashed curve). The density values are multiplied by 1000, and the smoothing parameter was set to 10^7.

individual distributions since, within each sample, there are children who are systematically fast and others who are systematically slow.

Figure 5.3 displays estimated ADHD density functions for selected individuals. We see that there is indeed considerable interchild variation in their shapes. The upper-left panel indicates more fast reactions than average, but a nearly uniform distribution of times beyond one second. The lower-left panel has a density more typical of control children, with no appreciably long tail. Both the right panels show a pronounced secondary mode to the right of one second, and the bottom panel even has a slight tertiary mode.

5.3   Estimating density and individual differences

The individual densities plotted in Figure 5.3 give us a visual impression that the ADHD children vary considerably among themselves in terms of their reaction-time distributions. This would be consistent, for example, with the presence of a disability that varied in severity. How can we represent the unusual shape of these reaction time distributions, and still give some indication of how these children vary?

A few critical remarks are in order about the usual way in which reaction-time data are analyzed. The nearly universal practice of using mean reaction time to represent a subject's typical performance has serious drawbacks. The first is that the mean is a much less appropriate measure of centrality when the distribution is strongly skewed than it is for nearly symmetric distributions like the normal. The long positive tail tends to pull the mean toward it and at the same time increase the variability of its estimate. The mode, by contrast, would be a better indication of a typical reaction time.

The other defect of the mean has to do with how it is modeled. Standard statistical tools such as analysis of variance and regression analysis postulate that whatever changes the typical reaction changes it *additively*. This amounts to saying that a little bit is added or subtracted to all reaction times by causal factors such as the presence of ADHD. But the results in Figure 5.2 suggest something more like a *multiplicative* impact of ADHD in which short reaction times are affected less than long reaction times, and leading, consequently, to the long positive tail being exaggerated. According to a multiplicative impact model, reaction times are affected by a percentage increase rather than a simple shift.

Let us explore, therefore, the variation from child to child and from group to group by using the following transformation for reaction time t measured in milliseconds,

$$z = \log_{10}(t - 120) . \tag{5.2}$$

The constant 120 is first subtracted because this is more like the true "zero" of reaction times, being about the fastest reaction time that is achievable. The log transformation of the shifted reaction times acknowledges that the impact of ADHD is more multiplicative than additive, and therefore that the impact on a logarithmic time scale will be more additive than it will be in the original time scale.

We may now propose the following additive model to describe the log transformed reaction time z_{ijk} of child i on trial j in group k:

$$z_{ijk} = \mu_k + \alpha_{i|k} + U_{ijk} . \tag{5.3}$$

The parameter μ_k quantifies the typical performance of children in group k and the parameter $\alpha_{i|k}$, read "child i within group k," quantifies the individual typical performance of this child. As is usual in ANOVA models, we fix the relative sizes of these effects by imposing the restriction

$$\sum_{i=1}^{N_k} \alpha_{i|k} = 0,$$

where N_k is the number of children in group k.

The residual term U_{ijk} expresses the lack of fit of the model for a specific reaction time, and it is the variation of the values of U_{ijk} that we see in

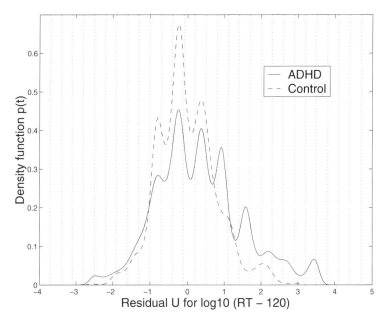

Figure 5.4. The densities of log-shifted reaction-time residuals U_{ijk} for 17 ADHD or hyperactive children (solid line) and 16 normal children (dashed line). Mean effects for individual control children have been removed, so that this group's density is centered on 0. The ADHD density is centered on 0.33 (corresponding to 122 msec) in order to emphasize the coherence of the modes. The vertical dotted lines indicate the knot placement in the B-spline basis described in Section 5.6.

the distribution of transformed reaction times for a specific child. We are assuming that this variable has a mean of zero. If we want to express what model (5.3) means for reaction time itself, then we can reverse the transformation (5.2) to get

$$\tau_i = 120 + 10^{\mu_k + \alpha_{i|k} + U_{ijk}} \ .$$

But can we be so sure that the distribution of the residuals U_{ijk} is normal? Not at all. We will want to preserve the idea of nonparametric estimation of the density function $p_k(u)$, where the subscript k indicates that we allow the distribution to be different for the two groups. Our technique for estimating these densities starts from that used to estimate the densities in Figures 5.2 and 5.3, but adds the capacity to estimate the model components μ_k and $\alpha_{i|k}$ in addition.

The estimated densities for the residuals for the two groups in this experiment are displayed in Figure 5.4. We see that the hyperactive children show greater variability in residuals U_{ijk}, even after the shifted log transformation, and we also see that the transformed times remain somewhat positively skewed. The mean μ_1 of the ADHD group was 2.92, corresponding to 952 msec, and the control mean μ_2 was 2.72, or 645 msec. As expected, this difference was highly significant ($t = 4.8$).

The pattern of modes in the two densities is striking. We can see this level of detail in the group densities because individual effects have been removed by estimating the individual shift parameters $\alpha_{i|k}$. In the plot, the center of the ADHD density has been shifted by what is equivalent to about 120 msec to show how well lined up the modes are. Initially, there was a suggestion that this multimodal behavior pointed to a substantive feature of brain function. On reflection, however, the experimenters realized that it was an artifact of the instrumentation, which gave some preference to times on particular cycles. Although this conclusion is not as exciting as the neurophysiological one, it illustrates the way in which statistical analyses can be important in drawing experimenters' attention to aspects they had previously overlooked.

5.4   Exploring variation across subjects with PCA

For each child, the work described in Section 5.3 yields an estimated density function for the log-shifted reaction times z for that child. This density function can be regarded as a functional datum for that child. In this section, we explore the use of functional principal components analysis to get a sense of how the density functions vary from child to child, and how many substantial components of variation there are. In Section 5.2, we only looked at an elementary aspect of this variation, namely a variation only in the center of the distributions. As we have seen in previous chapters, PCA offers the possibility of uncovering modes of variation that are more complex. As in Section 5.2, we work with the density functions $p_i(z)$ for log-shifted reaction times z defined in (5.3). We look only at the ADHD group.

Principal components analysis is not well adapted to describing variation in constrained functions. This is because principal components analysis provides an expansion of the data in terms of empirically defined basis functions, namely the principal components weight functions or *harmonics*. Thus there is no convenient way to ensure that the approximation of a density based on these harmonics will remain nonnegative. Instead of analyzing the densities directly, therefore, we study the variation in the *derivatives* of the functions $W_i(z)$ defined in (5.1), that is, the log-density derivative functions

$$w_i(z) = \frac{d}{dz} W_i(z) = \frac{d}{dz} \log p_i(z) \ .$$

One feature that makes these functions interesting is that, for the normal distribution, $w_i(z)$ is a straight line with negative slope. We can, therefore,

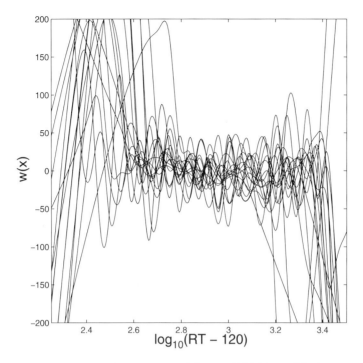

Figure 5.5. Log-density derivatives $w_i(z) = (d/dz) \log p_i(z)$ for individual log-shifted reaction-time densities for the 17 ADHD children.

investigate departures from normality such as multimodality by seeing how different these functions are from linear.

Figure 5.5 shows what these functions look like for the ADHD children. We confess that at first glance they do not look promising. But note that between about $z = 2.75$ and $z = 3.25$, there is something of a linear trend. Outside this central region, however, there is little if any structure visible. However, all the densities themselves are near zero outside the region [2.75, 3.25], and we are not particularly interested in what the functions $w_i(z)$ are up to over values of z that are extremely unlikely to occur. Therefore we use a weighted version of PCA, with weight the average density $\bar{p}(z)$ for the sample. This choice of weight diminishes the role of variation in $w_i(z)$ in defining the harmonics when the density itself is small. The weighted PCA proceeds by applying a standard PCA to the functions $\bar{p}(z)^{1/2} w_i(t)$. Once the harmonics $\eta_m(z)$ are identified for this analysis, we then back-transform to compute the weighted-PCA harmonics $\xi_m(z) = \bar{p}(z)^{-1/2} \eta_m(z)$ for the original log density derivative functions $w_i(z)$.

The first three harmonics account for 63% of the variation in this weighted PCA. This seems reasonable, considering the amount of variability that we see in Figure 5.5. Figure 5.6 indicates that the first three log eigenvalues are noticeably larger than the linear trend in the remainder.

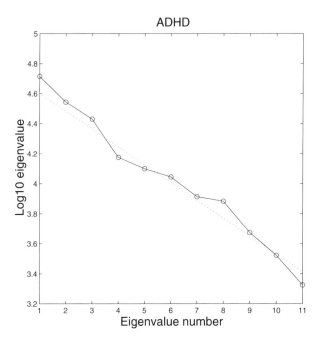

Figure 5.6. The logarithms of the eigenvalues for the weighted principal components analysis of the log-density derivative functions $w_i(z)$ for the ADHD children. The dotted line shows the linear trend for the log eigenvalues from 4 to 11.

Because of the density estimation context, we display the principal components or harmonics as effects on the mean density for the group by adding a multiple of the harmonic to the mean log density, and then converting this perturbed function to a density. The results for the first three principal components for the ADHD sample after varimax rotation are given in Figure 5.7. In each panel the density corresponding to the mean log-density derivative function $\bar{w}(z)$ is plotted as a dashed line for reference purposes.

The first harmonic mainly affects the height of the central peak of the distribution at the expense of moderate deviations from the peak. The second harmonic adds weight in the part of the distribution corresponding to very fast reaction times. The third harmonic corresponds to a density very much like the mean, but with the isolation of the three modes more sharply defined. This harmonic quantifies the strength of the quasiperiodic effect induced by the instrumentation in the experiment. These three harmonics all account for nearly equal amounts of variation.

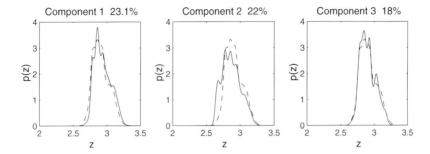

Figure 5.7. The effects of the first three varimax-rotated harmonics for the weighted principal components analysis of the log-density derivative functions $w_i(z)$ for the ADHD children. The solid line in each panel is the density resulting from adding a multiple of a harmonic to the mean function $\bar{w}(z)$ for the entire sample, and the dashed line is the density corresponding to the mean function $\bar{w}(z)$ itself.

5.5   What have we seen?

The effects of a disorder such as ADHD on a marker variable such as reaction time can be complex. These may go beyond a simple change of their central tendency to change the shape of the distribution itself. If we only use distributions that can change in simple ways, such as the normal which can change in location and scale only, we may miss some of these important distributional shape changes, and may at the same time get a distorted picture of simple shifts in distribution. In this case, we see that ADHD seems to create a long positive tail in addition to shifting the mode. Indeed, the strength of this tail seems to be an important component of variation, suggesting that perhaps the upper tail is the true marker for the severity of the ADHD condition.

An additional feature of our analysis was its ability to highlight the quasiperiodic behavior caused by the instrumentation; not only was this visible in the mean curves for the two populations, but one of the principal components was able to quantify the strength of the effect.

The statistical technology that makes our analyses possible is the nonparametric estimation of a density function, whether $p(t)$ for the reaction times, $p(z)$ for the log-shifted reaction times, or $p(u)$ for the residuals in model (5.3). Our method is not the only one available, and kernel density estimation is an alternative approach that is better known. However, our method of estimating the log density leads naturally into using the derivatives of the log densities as functional data for further analysis.

5.6   Technical details

When studying a density function like $p(t)$, we expand the function $W(t) = \text{constant} + \log p(t)$ in a B-spline basis, as described in Section 2.5, to give the expansion

$$W(x) = \sum_{k=1}^{K} c_k B_k(x). \tag{5.4}$$

There is no restriction on the values of the coefficients c_k. In the work described in this chapter, we used 34 B-spline basis functions of order 5, with equally spaced knots. Splines of order 5 were used so we would be able to define roughness penalties based on high derivatives, and to ensure that the derivative of $W(x)$ was itself smooth.

Given a sample $t_1, \ldots, t_N$ modeled by the density function $p(t)$, the density is estimated using a penalized maximum likelihood method proposed by Silverman (1982). The method applies a penalty on the roughness of $W(t)$ by maximizing the penalized log likelihood criterion

$$\text{PENMLE} = \sum_i \ln p(t_i) + \lambda \int_{t_L}^{t_U} W'''(u)^2 \, du \ . \tag{5.5}$$

There are two reasons for penalizing the integrated squared third derivative of the function $W(t)$. We use the derivative $w(t) = W'(t)$ for further analysis, and the penalty expressed in terms of w is the more familiar integrated squared second derivative. In addition, the penalty will be zero if and only if $W(t)$ is a quadratic function, which corresponds to $p(t)$ being a normal density (truncated over the interval of interest). Thus, if the smoothing λ increased without limit, it would force $W(t)$ to be quadratic and consequently $p(t)$ to be the normal density, which is the standard "parametric" density estimate.

To carry out the procedure numerically, the function $W(t)$ is expanded in terms of coefficients c_k as in (5.4), and the log likelihood,

$$\ln L = \sum_i \ln p(t_i)$$

and its first two derivatives are expressed in terms of the function $W(t)$ as

$$\ln L = \sum_{i=1}^{N} W(t_i) - N \ln \int \exp[W(u)]du$$

$$D_c \ln L = \sum_{i=1}^{N} D_c W(t_i) - N\text{E}[D_c W]$$

$$D_c^2 \ln L = \sum_{i=1}^{N} D_c^2 W(t_i) - N\text{E}[D_c^2 W] - N \text{Var}[D_c W],$$

where the notations D_c and D_c^2 mean taking the first and second partial derivatives with respect to c, respectively. Also, $\mathrm{E}[W] = \int W(u)g(u)\,du$, and similarly for $\mathrm{E}[D_cW]$ and $\mathrm{E}[D_c^2W]$. The values of the integrals in these expressions were approximated using numerical methods rather than analytically.

We use the method of scoring, which is defined by replacing the second derivative matrix in the Newton–Raphson method by $-N\,\mathrm{Var}[D_cW(t)]$. Convergence is rapid and stable in our experience. The computation is made simpler if $W(t_L)$ is zero, a condition that is easily assured if we fix the coefficient c_1 to zero for the first B-spline basis function, which is the only basis function that is nonzero at t_L.

When applying the method, the smoothing parameter values were chosen subjectively. Where the data are pooled across children, as in Figure 5.2, we used the value $\lambda = 10^6$. Where individual children are considered, and the sample size is smaller, the variability is larger and so a larger value of the smoothing parameter is appropriate. For example, in Figure 5.3, the value was $\lambda = 10^7$.

Software and further details are available from the Web page corresponding to this chapter.

6
Zooming in on Human Growth

6.1 Introduction

The careful documentation of human growth is essential in order to define what we call normal growth, so that we can detect as early as possible when something is going wrong with the growth process. Auxologists, the scientists that specialize in the study of growth, also need high quality data to advance our understanding of how the body regulates its own growth. It may come as a surprise to learn that human growth at the macro level that we see in our children is not that well understood.

Growth data are exceedingly expensive to collect since children must be brought into the laboratory at preassigned ages over about a 20-year span. Meeting this observational regime requires great dedication and persistence by the parents, and the dropout rate is understandably high, even taking for granted the long-term commitment of maintaining a growth laboratory. The Fels Institute in Ohio, for example, has been collecting growth data since 1929, and is now measuring the third generation for some of its original cases.

The accurate measurement of height is also difficult, and requires considerable training. Height diminishes throughout the day as the spine compresses, but it also depends on other factors. Infants must be measured lying down, and when the transition is made to measuring their standing height, measurements shrink by around one centimeter. The most careful procedures still exhibit standard deviations over repeated measurements of about three millimeters.

Records of a child's height over 20 years display features, described below, that are difficult for a data analyst to model. The classic approach has been to use mathematical functions depending on a limited number of unknown constants, and auxologists have shown much ingenuity in developing these parametric models to capture these features. The best models have eight or more parameters, and are still viewed as possibly missing some aspects of actual growth.

Nonparametric modeling techniques developed over the last three decades, such as kernel and spline smoothing methods, have been applied to growth data. These methods have been successful at detecting new features missed by parametric models, but they are not guaranteed to produce smoothing curves that are monotonic, or strictly increasing. Even a small failure of monotonicity in a height curve can have serious consequences for the corresponding growth velocity, and even more so for acceleration curves, which are especially important in identifying processes regulating growth.

In this chapter we look at some new developments in growth data analysis. A recently developed method for monotonic smoothing is applied to some old and new data. This method is used for all the curves estimated below, and is described in Section 6.8.3. Another aspect of the analysis is the introduction of *curve registration* methods, which allow the separation of amplitude and phase variation.

6.2   Height measurements at three scales

Figure 6.1 shows, for each of 10 girls, the height function $H(t)$ as estimated from 31 observations taken between 1 and 18 years. These data were collected as part of the Berkeley Growth Study; for more details of these data, and the other data analyzed in detail in this chapter, see Section 6.8.2. Growth is the most rapid in the earliest years, but we note the increase in slope during the pubertal growth spurt (PGS) that occurs at ages ranging from about 9 to 15 years. One girl is tall for all ages, but some girls can be tall during childhood, but end up with a comparatively small adult stature. The intervals between height measurements are six months or more, and the picture from this long-term perspective is of a relatively smooth growth process.

Figure 6.2 zooms in on growth by using measurements of a boy's height at 83 days over one school year, with gaps corresponding to the school vacations. The measurement noise in the data, of standard deviation about 3 mm, is apparent. The trend is also noticeably more bumpy, with height increasing more rapidly over some weeks than others.

To zoom in further, more accurate measurements are essential. The length of the tibia of a baby measured to within about 0.1 mm is graphed

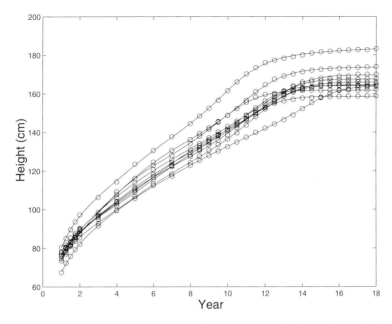

Figure 6.1. The heights of the first 10 females in the Berkeley Growth Study. Circles indicate the ages at which measurements were taken.

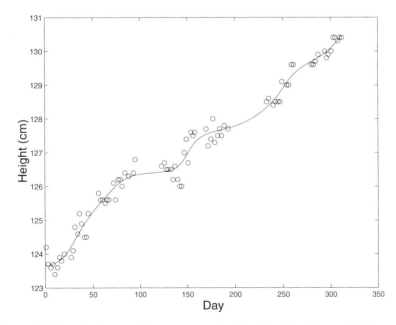

Figure 6.2. The circles are 83 measurements of height of a 10-year-old boy, and the solid curve is a smooth monotone fit to the data, as described in Section 6.8.3.

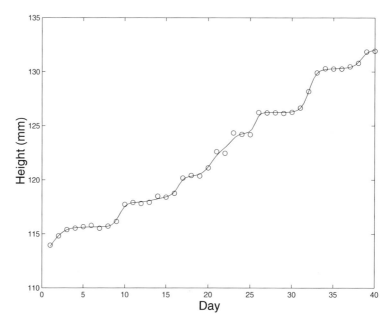

Figure 6.3. The dots indicate lengths of the tibia in the lower leg of a newborn infant, and the solid curve is a smooth monotone estimate of height.

in Figure 6.3. The jumps, or saltations, that we saw in the boy's growth are now much more visible. These data demand that we find a way to estimate just how much bone length changes over, say, a 24-hour period. Since bone length can only increase, it is essential that any smooth line, such as that in the figure, also be everywhere increasing, and this is one of the features of the smoothing method we use.

6.3   Velocity and acceleration

Although we commonly refer to data and curves such as shown in these figures as "growth curves," the term growth really means change. Hence, it is the velocity function $V(t)$, the instantaneous rate of change in height at time t, that is the real growth curve, and we should use the term "growth" to mean $V(t)$. Because height does not decrease (at least during the growing years), velocity or growth is necessarily positive. The height data only indirectly reflect growth, because they are measures of the *consequences* of growth.

If height observations are taken at time points t_i, we might consider estimating velocity by the difference ratio,

$$V(t_i) = [H(t_{i+1}) - H(t_i)]/(t_{i+1} - t_i),$$

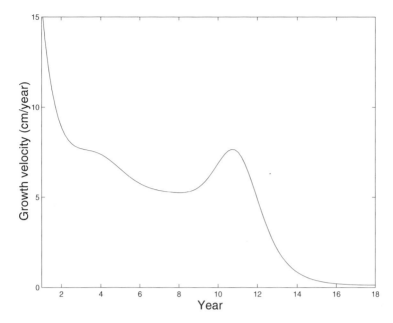

Figure 6.4. The estimated growth velocity, or rate of growth, of the first girl whose data are in Figure 6.1.

but this a bad idea from a statistical perspective, since even a small amount of noise in the height measurements will have a huge effect on the ratio, and this problem only gets worse as the time points get closer together. It is much better to fit the height data with an appropriate smooth curve, and then estimate velocity by finding the slope of this smooth curve.

Figures 6.4 through 6.6 display estimated velocity curves for the long-, medium-, and short-term growth examples considered above. Now we can see much more clearly what is happening. The pubertal spurt in Figure 6.4 is certainly more obvious, but even more impressive are the velocity surges for the 10-year-old boy. The peaks in velocity for the baby, exceeding two millimeters per day, are simply astonishing. We now know that we need to work hard to get good methods for estimating velocity, which at least during infancy is revealed to be a very intricate process.

We can get more understanding of the growth process by studying the rate of change in velocity; this is the *acceleration* in height, denoted by $A(t)$. Estimated acceleration curves for the 10 girls in the Berkeley data are given in Figure 6.7. Now we can see even more clearly what happens in the pubertal growth spurt. Naturally there is a big positive surge in velocity at the beginning of the PGS, followed by a return to zero when the velocity is no longer increasing, and finally a negative change in velocity in the final phase. It can be seen that the timing of the pubertal growth spurt varies a great deal from one girl to another, a feature we return to in

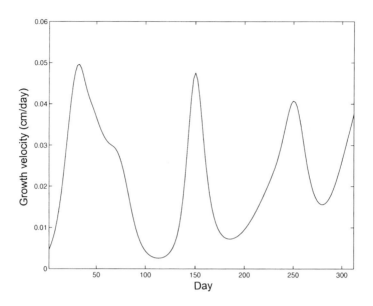

Figure 6.5. The estimated growth velocity of the boy whose data are in Figure 6.2.

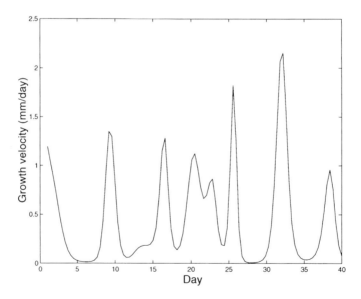

Figure 6.6. The estimated growth velocity of the baby whose data are in Figure 6.3.

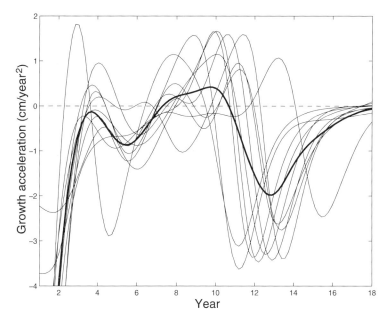

Figure 6.7. The estimated growth acceleration curves for the 10 girls whose data are shown in Figure 6.1. The heavy solid line is the average of these 10 curves.

Section 6.5. But what can also be seen, for several girls, are one or more smaller oscillations in acceleration before the pubertal growth spurt. The capacity to detect these so-called *midspurts* was one of the important early achievements of nonparametric curve estimation technology in this area.

6.4 An equation for growth

What causes the velocity $V(t_i)$ at age t_i to change to $V(t_{i+1})$ for the next observation time t_{i+1}? The question can be formulated by the following equation,

$$V(t_{i+1}) - V(t_i) = w_i V(t_i)(t_{i+1} - t_i). \qquad (6.1)$$

This equation is not a model for growth, but merely a way of looking at it. It relates the velocity change over the interval $t_{i+1} - t_i$ to three factors.

- $t_{i+1} - t_i$ itself. The smaller this time interval, the less change there will be, and in the limit $\Delta t \to 0$, velocity will not change. This says that over very small time scales growth is essentially a smooth process, an assertion that seems beyond question since a jump in the rate of growth over an arbitrarily small time interval would seem inconceivable in terms of the body's physiology.

- $V(t_i)$, a term that measures growth changes on a percentage or relative basis. This is particularly useful in allowing for variations in height over the population, and, for instance, allows for comparison of growth patterns independently of people's ultimate adult height.

- w_i, a factor that determines the change in velocity. We make this factor depend on t_i because we imagine that this factor itself will change with time. This is the factor that really specifies how growth varies.

Asking a question in the right way is everything in science, and the formulation in (6.1) focuses our attention on the size of the factor w_i, which will be positive if velocity is increasing at age t_i, zero if there is no change, and negative if velocity is decreasing.

Here is a rearrangement of equation (6.1):

$$\frac{V(t_{i+1}) - V(t_i)}{t_{i+1} - t_i} = w_i V(t_i). \tag{6.2}$$

The left side of this equation is just an estimate of the instantaneous rate of change of $V(t)$, and becomes the acceleration $A(t)$ when $t_{i+1} - t_i \to 0$. Therefore, rather than defining w_i to satisfy (6.1) and (6.2) exactly, we replace it by a function $w(t)$ defined by

$$A(t) = w(t)V(t) \quad \text{or} \quad w(t) = \frac{A(t)}{V(t)}. \tag{6.3}$$

The continuously defined function $w(t)$ is now the ratio of acceleration to velocity, or what we can call *relative acceleration*, meaning acceleration of height measured as a fraction of velocity. We can rewrite (6.3) as the differential equation

$$\frac{d^2 H}{dt^2} = w(t)\frac{dH}{dt}. \tag{6.4}$$

The general solution to this equation is

$$H(t) = C_0 + C_1 \int_0^t [\exp \int_0^u w(v)\, dv]\, du. \tag{6.5}$$

In this expression, C_0 and C_1 are arbitrary constants that will need to be estimated from data.

Equation (6.4) may be described as the fundamental equation of growth, in the sense that any intrinsically smooth growth process may be expressed in this way. The relative acceleration $w(t)$ is the *functional parameter of growth*. Our approach to thinking about growth is to model this function, rather than the height function itself. Once we have a way of estimating $w(t)$, we can check it against the data by using equation (6.5). To see how we estimate $w(t)$, go to Section 6.8.3.

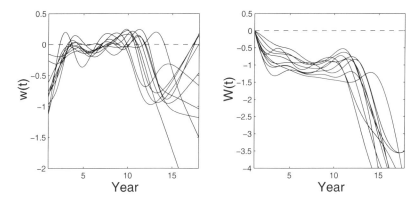

Figure 6.8. The left panel shows the relative acceleration function $w(t)$, and the right panel its integral $W(t)$.

For the 10 girls we have been studying, Figure 6.8 displays the functions $w(t)$, as well as their integrals

$$W(t) = \int_0^t w(u)du \; . \tag{6.6}$$

It can be shown from (6.5) that $W(t)$ is proportional to $\log H'(t)$, the logarithm of the instantaneous growth rate. We see that $w(t)$ looks rather like the acceleration curves in Figure 6.7 except at the end in late adolescence. This is a consequence of $w(t)$ being relative acceleration, as expressed in equation (6.3).

6.5   Timing or phase variation in growth

As in any data analysis, important aims for the long-term growth data are to estimate the average features of growth, and to get an impression of their variability across individuals. However, Figure 6.7 shows that these tasks, which are straightforward for univariate and multivariate data, present a new challenge. The heavy line, which is the mean of the 10 acceleration curves, does not have the characteristics of any of the observed curves. The PGS peak and valley for the average are much too small, but on the other hand the duration of the PGS for the average curve is longer than that of any single observed curve.

The problem is that the growth curves exhibit two types of variability. *Amplitude* variability pertains to the sizes of particular features such as the velocity peak in the pubertal growth spurt, ignoring their timings. *Phase* variability is variation in the timings of the features without considering their sizes. Before we can get a useful measure of a typical growth curve, we must separate these two types of variation, so that features such as the

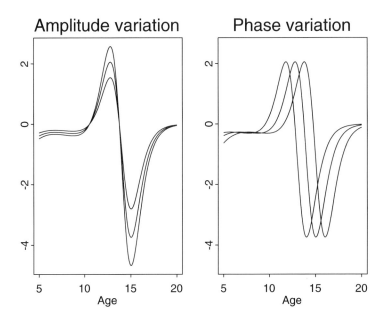

Figure 6.9. The left panel shows three height acceleration curves varying only in amplitude. The right panel shows three curves varying only in phase.

pubertal spurt occur at roughly the same "times" for all girls. The problem is expressed in schematic terms in Figure 6.9, where we see in the left panel two acceleration curves that differ only in amplitude, and in the right panel two curves with the same amplitude, but differing in phase.

By "time" here we now mean something like physiological time, which need not unfold at the same rate as physical or clock time. We mean that two girls in the middle of the pubertal spurt are, effectively, at the same physiological age, whatever their respective chronological ages. What we need is some way of mapping clock time t into its physiological counterpart. That is, we want a function $h_i(t)$ for girl i such that at physiological time t this girl has a chronological age of $h_i(t)$. For example, if $h(t) > t$, we have someone who is growing late, and if t is the physiological age at which the growth spurt takes place, then this person is having the PGS at a clock age that is later. The curve $h(t)$ is often called a *time warping* function. Figure 6.10 displays these functions $h(t)$ for our 10 girls. Remember that curves above the diagonal correspond to late growth, and curves below the diagonal to early growth.

But isn't time, too, a positive growth process? It always increases because days and years accumulate, and its velocity is defined by the time units that we use. Or at least, that is so for clock time, which increases linearly, corresponding to relative acceleration $w(t) = 0$. But physiological time, which is driven by factors such as hormonal secretions that are not constant

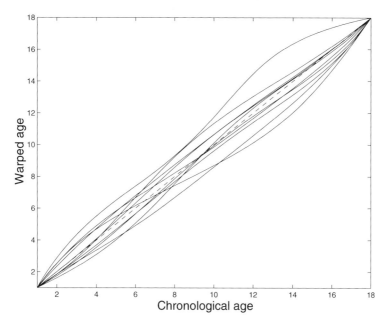

Figure 6.10. The time warping functions $h(t)$ for the 10 Berkeley girls. Curves above the diagonals indicate girls with a physiological age consistently earlier than chronological age, and therefore growing late.

across individuals, need not unfold in this elementary way. Even in Figure 6.1 we can see clearly that some girls are outstripping clock time, and maturing early, while other girls are lagging behind the clock, being late maturers.

Therefore, the warping function $h(t)$, which must be always increasing, reflects simply another type of growth curve, and may be characterized by the same mathematical representation that we have in equation (6.4), and therefore corresponds to its own relative acceleration $w_h(t)$. We defer further details on how we estimate $h(t)$ to Chapter 7, where registration is the main topic, and pass to what we see when the growth curves have been registered.

6.6   Amplitude and phase variation in growth

What do we do with warping functions $h_i(t)$ once we have estimated them? Recalling that for a late grower, $h(t) > t$, we see that we can think of $h(t)$ in such a case as "speeding up" clock time to make it match physiological time. This means that if we calculate the function

$$V^*(t) = V[h(t)] \tag{6.7}$$

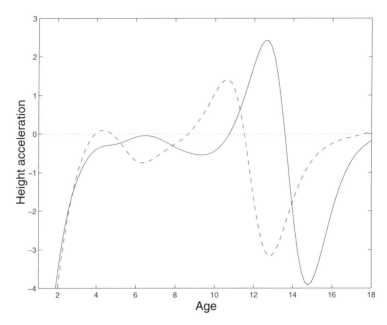

Figure 6.11. The solid curve is the average acceleration for the registered data from the boys, and the dashed curve is the registered acceleration average for the girls.

we now have a new velocity function $V^*(t)$ that shows the pubertal growth spurt, for example, as occurring at the "right time." Similarly, for $h(t) < t$, we can use the warping function to slow down clock time for an early grower. We also define the registered height and acceleration curves $H^*(t) = H[h(t)]$ and $A^*(t) = A[h(t)]$, respectively.

With these registered curves in hand, we can now carry out averaging and other analyses more meaningfully, since registered curves no longer have the phase variation that affected the average in Figure 6.7. Figure 6.11 superimposes the mean registered acceleration curves of girls and boys. Some new features now emerge. We see that the pubertal spurt is not the only spurt visible in long-term growth data, and we already know that there are even more spurts within medium- and short-term data.

We see in Figure 6.11 that girls and boys seem to go through the same pubertal growth cycles, but differ in two ways: the PGS is earlier in girls, but more intense in boys. The time shift prompts us to warp time for one gender in order to render its growth equivalent to the other. The left panel of Figure 6.12 displays the warping function $h(t)$ that registers the boys' data to the girls', and the right panel shows the registered average acceleration curves. We can see two major gender differences. The left panel demonstrates that male growth essentially lags behind female growth, with a gap that increases steadily until growth is finally finished. The right panel

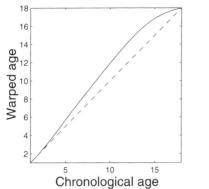
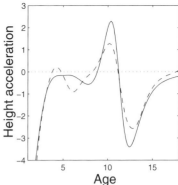

Figure 6.12. The left panel displays the warping function for registering the boys' average velocity to that of the girls. Because boys mature more slowly, the warping function is above the diagonal, shown as a dashed line. The right panel shows the registered average acceleration curves. The solid curve corresponds to the boys and the dashed curve to the girls.

shows that the intensity of the acceleration function during the pubertal spurt is greater for boys than for girls. These are the two main contributors to the gender difference in mean adult heights: boys grow over a longer period, and grow more intensely during the pubertal growth spurt.

The right panel of Figure 6.12 also shows some gender difference in earlier childhood. Closer examination of these data, and also of other larger data sets on growth such as the Fels Institute data, reveals that many children have more than one midspurt. Furthermore, both the number and the registered position of these midspurts is more variable in boys than in girls. This is partly because boys have a longer prepubertal period. It is the averaging out of this greater intergender variability that causes boys to have a flatter average registered acceleration curve.

What of the amplitude variation among the girls? A functional principal components analysis of the registered acceleration reveals that three principal components or harmonics account for 72% of their variation about the mean acceleration curve. After varimax rotation of these components, we get the three components displayed in Figure 6.13, and they account for nearly equal proportions of variance. Varimax harmonic 1 has to do only with variation during the pubertal spurt, and therefore captures the intensity of this event. The second and third harmonics, on the other hand, reflect variation only in the prepubertal years, but rather differently. The second harmonic shows an intensification of the two prepubertal spurts relative to the mean curve, but the third is more complex, capturing phase variation in these two earlier spurts that was not taken out by the registration process.

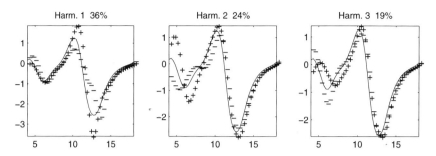

Figure 6.13. The varimax-rotated harmonics of registered acceleration for the girls. The amount of variation accounted for is indicated at the top of each harmonic. The solid curve is the mean acceleration, and the plus and minus symbols show the effects of adding and subtracting a multiple of the harmonic to the mean.

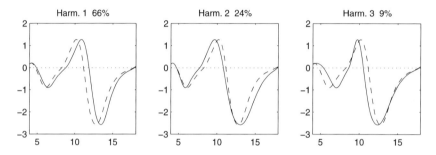

Figure 6.14. Results of a PCA of the warping functions, regarded as functional data in their own right. The dashed curves show the mean acceleration curve without time transformation, and the solid curves show what the mean acceleration curve would look like under the influence of each harmonic. The underlying data are the growth data for the 10 females in the Berkeley growth study.

We can also study phase variation by carrying out a PCA of the warping functions in Figure 6.10. The harmonics are displayed in Figure 6.14 by showing what the mean acceleration would look like if a multiple of the harmonic were added to clock time. In this case, the first three components explain 99% variation. The first harmonic corresponds to growth that is consistently late. The second shows early growth up to the deceleration phase of the PGS, and then slow recovery. The third indicates late prepubertal growth and early onset of puberty.

6.7 What we have seen?

Growth is not at all smooth over a short time scale. Our results hint that growth takes place by turning on and off the velocity function periodically.

In an infant the period is three or four days, but later the period seems to lengthen, until by 10 years it is of the order of a number of weeks. The discovery of these jumps or saltations is new, and we need much more data of the quality that we have for the baby before we can understand this process better. But perhaps what counts for growth is what turns it off; growth at the rate displayed in Figure 6.6 could actually be dangerous if sustained for much longer than a day or so.

On the methodological side, a formulation of the growth process in terms of the difference equation (6.1) or the differential equation (6.4) leads to a smoothing technology for growth data that respects the monotonicity of the height function $H(t)$ and the positivity of velocity $V(t)$, and also yields in the form of relative acceleration $w(t)$ a curve with a natural interpretation. An added bonus was the appreciation that the time warping function $h(t)$ that takes clock time into physiological time is also a growth process, and this story is taken up further in Chapter 7. The time warping functions for each individual can themselves be considered as functional data.

Finally, once we have teased apart, at least to some extent, amplitude and phase variation, we see that boys and girls do not differ strikingly in the shapes of their acceleration amplitudes, but that they do show a large amount of phase variation. Among the girls (and boys as well), amplitude variation seems to be primarily three-dimensional, and separable into components that reflect variation in the pubertal growth spurt, and others that show variation in prepubertal growth.

6.8   Notes and further issues

6.8.1   Bibliography

The work of this chapter is discussed in more detail in Ramsay and Bock (2002). They provide extensions and more details of the analyses presented here, apply the methods to the larger Fels Institute data set, and give further discussion and bibliographic references. The formulation of the growth process as a second-order linear differential equation, and the analysis of the growth data for the 10-year-old boy, are given in Ramsay (1998). The companion paper, Ramsay and Li (1998), applies this formulation to the registration problem, which is examined in more detail in Chapter 7.

There is already a large literature containing functional data analyses of growth data. Indeed, this field has provided one of the most important test beds for the development of curve estimation and analysis. The many contributions of T. Gasser and his collaborators, of which Gasser et al. (1990) is only one example, are especially important. A good deal of the research in this fascinating field appears in *Annals of Human Biology*.

Growth curve analysis has also inspired many contributions to the curve registration problem, and statistical issues in the use of features or landmarks to register growth curves has been studied by Kneip and Gasser (1992) and Gasser and Kneip (1995).

6.8.2   The growth data

The Berkeley Growth Study (Tuddenham and Snyder, 1954) recorded the heights of 54 girls and 39 boys between the ages of 1 and 18 years. Although larger studies of growth have since been completed, notably the Fels (Roche, 1992) and Zurich (Falkner, 1960) data, the Berkeley data have been published and are therefore freely available. Heights were measured at 31 ages for each child, and the standard error of these measurements was about 3 mm, tending to be larger in early childhood and lower in later years.

The data on the growth of the 10-year-old boy were collected as part of a study reported in Thalange et al. (1996), and generously made available to us by P. J. Foster at the University of Manchester. The short-term data on the growth of the tibia in a newborn infant are described in Hermanussen et al. (1998), and we thank Prof. Hermanussen for supplying them. This paper is one in a series of papers that provide details on the experimental procedure, and which report similar results in the growth of rats.

6.8.3   Estimating a smooth monotone curve to fit data

In this section, the monotone smoothing method is described briefly; for more details, see Ramsay (1998). Relevant software is available from the Web site corresponding to this chapter. We use the differential equation for growth $A(t) = w(t)V(t)$ to transform the problem of estimating the height function $H(t)$ that actually fits the height observations y_j observed at ages $t_j, j = 1, \ldots, n$ to one of estimating the relative acceleration function $w(t)$. Our task is made simpler by the fact that $w(t)$ is unconstrained in any way, unlike $V(t)$ which must be positive, or $H(t)$ which must always increase.

Our approach to estimating $w(t)$ is to express it as a linear combination of basis functions $\phi_k(t)$, as we already have done in previous chapters, so that

$$w(t) = \sum_{k=1}^{K} c_k \phi_k(t). \tag{6.8}$$

We can then fit the data by numerically minimizing the error sum of squares

$$\mathrm{SSE} = \sum_{j=1}^{n} [y_j - H(t_j)]^2 \tag{6.9}$$

with respect to the coefficients c_k defining the basis function expansion (6.8).

Our choice of basis is the B-spline basis $\phi_k(t) = B_k(t)$ described briefly in Section 2.5 and in detail in Ramsay and Silverman (1997, Chapters 3 and 4). We tend to choose this basis for any function that is not periodic and that has no other restrictions on its shape. A B-spline basis is defined by a set of knots, and our strategy is to place a knot at each age t_j at which height is observed.

Putting knots at every data point allows considerable flexibility, but results in more basis functions than there are observations. We compensate for this overly rich basis by adding a roughness penalty to the error sum of squares criterion (6.9) and then minimizing the following penalized least squares criterion

$$\text{PENSSE} = \sum_{j=1}^{n} [y_j - H(t_j)]^2 + \lambda \int_0^T [w''(t)]^2 dt. \qquad (6.10)$$

In this expression, T is the largest age at which we wish to estimate $H(t), V(t)$, and $A(t)$. Roughness in this expression is defined as the integral of the square of the second derivative $w''(t)$ of $w(t)$. Because of the nonlinear dependence of $H(t)$ on $w(t)$, the minimization of PENSSE will involve a numerical optimization over the vector of B-spline coefficients c_k.

The effect of varying the smoothing parameter λ in (6.10) is as follows. The closer λ is to zero, the less the roughness of $w(t)$ is penalized, and in the limit $H(t)$ will become a monotone curve that comes as close as any monotone curve can come to fitting the data, which, of course, may not be themselves strictly increasing. Such a curve is bound to have plateaus and points of very rapid increase, and would be unacceptable even for data as rough as those in Figure 6.3. At the other extreme, if λ were to increase without limit, $w(t)$ would approach a straight line, and $H(t)$ would become much too smooth to fit the data acceptably. In particular, $A(t)$ would become linear, and would not offer a plausible account of events such as the PGS. In the present context, we have found it satisfactory to choose subjectively the smallest value of λ that still provided a smooth and interpretable estimate of $A(t)$.

7

Time Warping Handwriting and Weather Records

7.1 Introduction

In Chapter 6 we encountered what is almost always a fact of life in functional data. Curves vary in two ways: vertically, so that certain oscillations and levels are larger in some curves than others; and horizontally, so that the timings or locations of prominent features in curves vary from curve to curve. We call these two types of variation *amplitude* and *phase*, respectively. You might want to glance back at Figure 6.9 to see a schematic diagram illustrating this concept.

We now look more closely at amplitude and phase variation in the context of two rather different sets of data. The first is a sample of the printing (by hand) of the characters "fda." Each observation is a series of strokes separated by gaps where the pen is lifted off the paper, along with the clock times associated with these events. The timing of strokes and cusps varies from sample to sample, and we consider how to register these curves by transforming time so that, as nearly as possible, each stroke occurs at the same time for all curves. The aim of registration is to yield a sample of curves that vary only in terms of amplitude. The phase variation does not disappear, though; it is captured in the time transformations that we estimate for each curve.

Our second example is a single long time series, daily temperature measurements for the 34 years spanning 1961 through 1994. Naturally these data have a strong annual pattern, but one has only to appeal to personal experience to know that winter, for example, arrives late in some years and early in others. Therefore, we want to speed up and slow down time within each year so that the seasons will change at the same time across all years. We do this for many reasons, among them to get a better estimate of the average annual temperature curve, and to get tighter estimates of long-term trends such as might be associated with global warming.

We reserve the discussion of the more technical aspects of just how registration is achieved to Section 7.6, but it will first be helpful to spell out more formally a model for how curves vary.

7.2   Formulating the registration problem

Curve registration can be expressed formally as follows. We have a sample of N functions x_i. Each curve is defined over an interval, and the length of the interval may vary from curve to curve. For simplicity, let us assume a common origin but a variable end point, and make the intervals $[0, T_i]$.

A basic form of registration is to preprocess each curve by rescaling its argument range to a common standard interval $[0, T_0]$. This standard time interval $[0, T_0]$ may, for example, be the average interval $[0, \bar{T}]$. Although we assume the existence of a standard interval, we do not require that the data have necessarily been scaled to fit this interval.

Now let $h_i(t)$ be a transformation of time t for curve i, which we call a *time warping function*. The argument t varies over $[0, T_0]$. The values of $h_i(t)$, however, range over the curve i's interval $[0, T_i]$, and satisfy the constraint $h_i(0) = 0$ and $h_i(T_0) = T_i$. Thus the time warping function maps the standard interval $[0, T_0]$ to the interval on which the function x_i lives.

The fact that the timings of events retain the same order regardless of the time scale implies that the time warping function h_i should be strictly increasing, so that $h_i(t_1) > h_i(t_2)$ if and only if $t_1 > t_2$. In fact, $h_i(t)$ is just a growth curve of the kind that we studied in Chapter 6. We can think of clock time t as growing linearly with a constant velocity of one second per second. We can think of curve i's "system time" as evolving at a rate that can change slightly from one clock unit to another. We show that printing is running ahead of itself at some times, and late at others; winter comes early some years, and late at others.

This strict monotonicity condition ensures that the function h_i is *invertible*, so that for each y in the interval $[0, T_i]$ there is a unique t for which $h(t) = y$. We use the notation h_i^{-1} to denote the inverse function,[1] for which $h_i^{-1}(y) = h_i^{-1}[h_i(t)] = t$. The invertibility of h_i means that it defines a one-to-one correspondence between the time points on the two different time scales.

---

[1] Not to be confused with the reciprocal of h, a concept which we do not use in this discussion.

Let $x_0(t)$ be a fixed function defined over $[0, T_0]$ that provides a template for the individual curves x_i in the sense that after registration, the features of x_i will be aligned in some sense to those of x_0. The following is a model for two functions $x_0(t)$ and $x_i(t)$ differing primarily in terms of phase variation,

$$x_i[h_i(t)] = x_0(t) + \epsilon_i(t) , \tag{7.1}$$

where the residual or disturbance function ϵ is small relative to x_i and roughly centered about 0. Because we assume that ϵ is small relative to x_i, this model postulates that major differences in shape between target function x_0 and specific function x_i are due only to phase variation. Having identified the N warping functions $h_i(t)$, we can then calculate the *registered functions* $x_i[h_i(t)]$. Methods for fitting the model (7.1) are developed later in this chapter.

What does $h(t)$ mean? Let's assume that the ice breaks up on the St. Lawrence River at Montreal on the average on April 7th, day 97 for nonleap years. But in 1975 spring is late and the ice goes out on April 14th, or day 104. We want, therefore, that $h_{1975}(97) = 104$, so that $x_{1975}[h_{1975}(97)] = x_{1975}(104)$, and therefore that, from a clock perspective, the ice is breaking up simultaneously in both the standard year and in 1975 when time is running a week late. In effect, in this case, the warping function speeds up time to compensate for its being tardy in 1975.

On the other hand, imagine that in the same year the leaves on Mont Royal in the city change color on September 15th (day 258) instead of September 30 (day 303) as is normal. Then $h_{1975}(303) = 258$, and the warping function is slowing down system time at a point when it is running ahead to conform to clock time. Thus, $h(t) > t$ corresponds to a process running slow, and $h(t) < t$ to one running fast.

In most of the examples we consider, the target function x_0 is not given. Instead we have to construct it from the data. Typically, we begin by mapping each interval linearly to the standard interval $[0, T_0]$, and set x_0 initially to be the sample mean $\bar{x}$ of the functions x_i after this scaling. We then register the individual functions to $\bar{x}$, and update the estimate of x_0 to be the mean of the *registered* functions. We now update the warping functions by registering the individual functions to this new estimate of x_0. In principle, it is possible to iterate the process of updating x_0 then reestimating the warping functions, but this is rarely necessary in practice.

The functions $x_i(t)$ that we are discussing here may be derivatives as, for example, the velocity curves in Chapter 6. It can be better to register derivatives instead of the original functions because derivatives tend to oscillate more, and therefore have more distinctive features to align. In addition, in phenomena such as human growth, features in the derivative are the true aspects of interest in the problem.

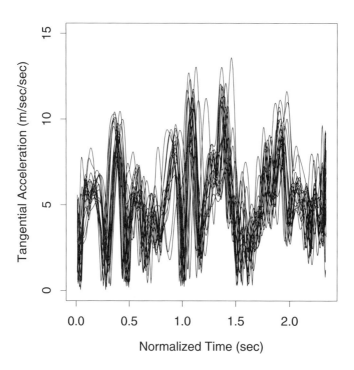

Figure 7.1. The tangential acceleration (7.2) on the X–Y plane for 20 samples of the printing of the characters "fda" by a single individual.

7.3 Registering the printing data

These data are recordings of the X-, Y-, and Z-coordinates 200 times per second of the tip of the pen during the printing by hand of the characters "fda." In the experiment, there were a number of subjects, and each repeated the printing 20 times. Because this is printing instead of cursive writing, the vertical Z-coordinate is important.

The registration problem is illustrated by plotting the magnitude of the *tangential acceleration* vector,

$$TA(t) = [X''(t) + Y''(t)]^{1/2} \qquad (7.2)$$

on the X–Y plane for each curve for one of our subjects. Tangential acceleration is an important property in the study of the dynamics of printing. To simplify the plot, the time taken to draw each record in Figure 7.1 was first normalized to the average time, 2.3 seconds. We see that the timings of the acceleration peaks vary noticeably from replication to replication.

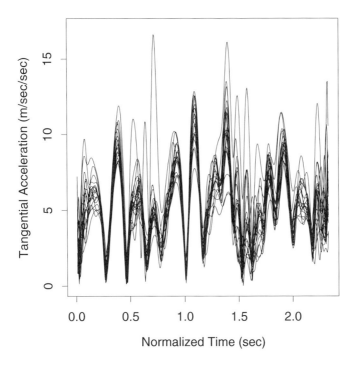

Figure 7.2. The tangential acceleration curves for the registered printing samples.

The registered results are shown in Figure 7.2, and we see that the acceleration peaks are now much more cleanly aligned. Moreover, when we look at the mean tangential acceleration calculated before and after registration, as shown in Figure 7.3, we see that the registration has also improved the amount of detail in the mean function. The peaks are higher, more sharply defined, the valleys are closer to zero, and some small peaks emerge that were washed out in the unregistered mean function.

We return to these data in Chapter 11, where we consider whether we can identify someone by using a differential equation that describes that person's printing.

7.4 Registering the weather data

Functional data often come to us as a single long time series spanning many days, months, years, or other time units. The variation in data such as these is usually multilevel in nature. There is usually a clear annual, diurnal, or other cycle over the basic time unit called the *season* of the data, combined

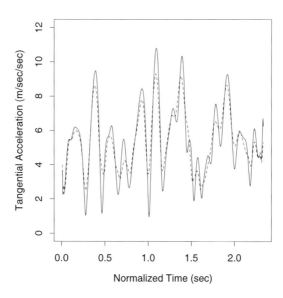

Figure 7.3. The mean tangential acceleration curve for the registered printing samples is plotted as a solid line, and the mean for the unregistered data as a dashed line.

with longer-term trends that span many time units. Moreover, the seasonal cycle may also show some evolution over the time spanned by the series.

The data in this example are 12,410 daily temperatures at Montreal over the 34 years from 1961 to 1994 (in leap years temperatures for February 28 and 29 were averaged). Because these are 24-hour averages, the actual daily lows and highs were more extreme. The minimum and maximum temperatures recorded in this period were $-30°$C and $30°$C, respectively. All our analyses are conducted on the entire series, but we do not *plot* the results for the entire time interval, since this is too much detail to put in a graph. Figure 7.4 focuses on 1989, when a severe cold snap came at Christmas, and was followed by a strong thaw.

We now smooth the temperatures in two ways. We smooth merely to remove the day-to-day variation, which from our perspective is too short-range to be interesting, although we are reluctant to call it error or noise. When we are done, we are left with an estimate of the smooth part of temperature variation. We achieved this by using 500 B-spline basis functions of order 6. The knots were equally spaced, and occurred at about every 25 days. This smooth, which we denote $x(t)$, is shown in Figure 7.4 as a solid line.

The second smooth $x_0(t)$ is designed to estimate the strictly periodic component of the sequence. This was achieved by expanding the series in

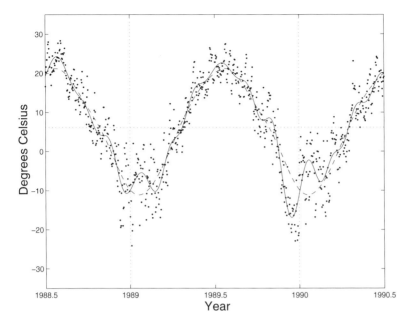

Figure 7.4. Temperature data for Montreal from mid-1988 to mid-1990. Daily mean temperatures are plotted as points, a smooth of the data as a solid line, and a strictly periodic trend as a dashed line. The horizontal dashed line indicates the mean temperature over the 34 years of data.

terms of nine Fourier basis functions with base period 365.25 days. In signal analysis jargon, we applied a high-pass filter. Now the standard deviation of the residuals from this trend was 4.74°C, which is necessarily higher than the unconstrained B-spline smooth, but we were surprised at how small the increase actually was. This periodic trend is shown as the dashed line in Figure 7.4.

We now subtract the strictly periodic curve $x_0(t)$ from the smooth curve $x(t)$ to highlight trends and events unexplained by seasonal variation. The result is shown in Figure 7.5, and the standard deviation of these differences is 2.15°C. We see the cold snap of 1989 as the strongest negative spike, and we also see a number of episodes where the smooth trend is either above or below zero for comparatively long periods. The temperature was higher than average for a long period after 1990, for example.

Some of this longer-term trend can be viewed as phase variation, due to the early or late arrival of some seasons. For example, the cold snap of 1989 would not have been so dramatic if it had come around January 15, 1990, when temperatures approaching −30°C happen more often, and indeed were seen a year earlier. We need to remove our estimate of the phase variation to get a better sense of just how extreme this event was.

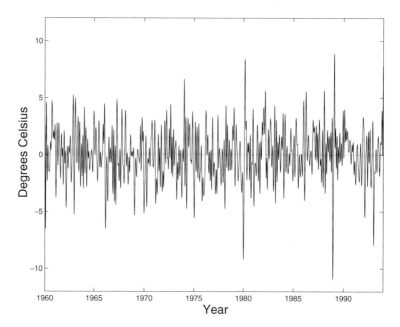

Figure 7.5. The difference between the smooth trend and the strictly periodic trend for the Montreal temperature data.

Figure 7.6 shows what happens around 1989 when we register the smooth trend $x(t)$ to the strictly periodic target $x_0(t)$. We used 140 B-spline basis functions of order 5 to define the relative acceleration function $w(t)$ defining time warping function $h(t)$ as described in Section 7.6, yielding a spacing between knots of three months. This seemed to give enough flexibility to capture some of the within-year phase variation, but not enough to distort fine features in the curves. Now we see that the cold snap at Christmas 1989 is positioned after registration in January 1990. The standard deviation of the differences between the registered temperature curve and the strictly periodic has now dropped to $1.73°$C. We can now estimate the proportion of the variation of the unconstrained smooth around the strictly periodic smooth due to phase variation by the squared multiple correlation $R^2 = (2.15^2 - 1.73^2)/2.15^2 = 0.35$. Thus, about a third of the smooth variation in temperature is due to phase.

To get some idea of how much shift in time is required to achieve the results in Figure 7.6, we can plot the difference between the warped and actual time functions $h(t) - t$, called the *time deformation function*. This is shown in Figure 7.7, and we see that midwinter in 1989/1990 arrived about 25 days early.

What about global warming? The smaller residuals for the registered data fit by strictly linear trend should help us to detect any long-term linear trend in the data. The slope for the regression of these residuals

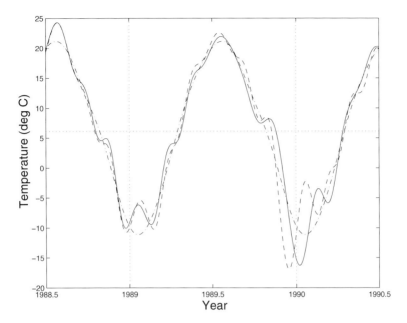

Figure 7.6. Temperature data for Montreal from mid-1988 to mid-1990 registered to the strictly periodic trend. The registered smooth of the data is the solid line, the unregistered smooth is the dashed line, and the strictly periodic trend is the dashed-dotted line. The horizontal dashed line indicates the mean temperature over the 34 years of data.

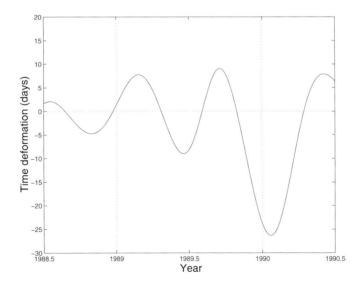

Figure 7.7. The time deformation function $h(t) - t$ for the registration results in Figure 7.6.

on time is 0.0024°C per year, a total of 0.08°C for the 34-year period of observation. The standard error of the regression coefficient, however, is 0.0016°C, and we cannot conclude that this amount of trend is significant.

7.5   What have we seen?

Although we have already seen the registration problem in Chapter 6, the two examples here introduce some new aspects. For the printing data we had to register the three coordinates simultaneously, that is, with a common time warping function $h(t)$. The amount of registration involved was substantially less than for the growth data, but we saw some rather dramatic improvements in the coherence of the tangential amplitude curves in Figure 7.2, and this turns out to be important when we analyze these data later.

Not all functional data involve multiple samples of curves. Rather, a long time series such as the temperature data also contains in a certain sense replicated data. There are 34 repetitions of the annual variation in temperature, and our strictly periodic smooth using the Fourier basis was, in fact, a type of averaging over these repetitions. When we registered the entire series to this periodic template, we discovered that the amount of phase variation was rather substantial, and required in certain years nearly a month of adjustment. Removing phase variation also led to a rather substantial reduction in the total variation of the smooth trend. This discovery seriously challenges most of the methods now used to analyze time series such as this, because they do not provide for phase variation.

7.6   Notes and references

In this section, we generally achieve some simplification of notation by dropping the subscript on the function $x_i(t)$ to be registered as well as the warping function $h_i(t)$.

7.6.1   Continuous registration

We may also register two curves by optimizing some measure of similarity of their shapes, and thus use the entire curves in the process. Put another way, the timings of a fixed set of landmarks provide one way of describing how similar the shapes of two curves are, but we can also choose measures that use the whole curves.

Silverman (1995) optimized a global fitting criterion with respect to a restricted parametric family of transformations of time shifts, and applied this approach to estimating a shift in time for each of the temperature

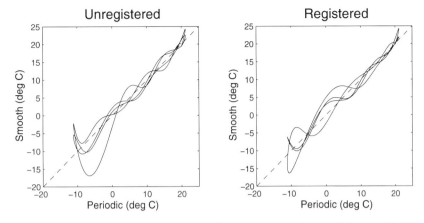

Figure 7.8. In the left panel the values of the unconstrained smooth from mid-1988 to mid-1990 are plotted against the corresponding values of the periodic smooth. In the right panel the registered smooth values are plotted against the periodic smooth values. We see that the values are now closer to the diagonal dashed line.

functions in 35 Canadian weather stations. He also incorporated this shift into a principal components analysis of the variation among curves, thus explicitly partitioning variation into range and domain components. His measure of shape similarity was the total squared error, cast into functional terms as

$$\text{FSSE}(h) = \int_0^{T_0} \{x[h(t)] - x_0(t)\}^2 \, dt \ . \tag{7.3}$$

This measure works well enough provided that the amount of amplitude variation is small, so that the pure phase variation model (7.1) is about right. However, the measure can run into trouble when $x(t)$ and $x_0(t)$ have the same shape but differ in amplitude. Ramsay and Li (1998) offer an example in which it is shown that this criterion has a tendency to "pinch in" the sides of the larger of the two curves in order to make it look more like the smaller.

To evolve an alternative fitting criterion, we could allow a scale factor A, which may depend on i, to yield

$$\text{FSSE}(h, A) = \int_0^{T_0} \{x[h(t)] - Ax_0(t)\}^2 \, dt \ . \tag{7.4}$$

This would be zero if $x_0(t)$ and $x[h(t)]$ differ only by a scale factor, so that $x(t) = Ax_0(t)$ for some positive constant A. This means that the two functions have essentially the same shape, and that the values of $x(t)$ are proportional to those of $x_0(t)$. If the curves are exactly proportional, then the matrix

$$\left[\begin{array}{cc} \int \{x_0(t)\}^2 \, dt & \int x_0(t)x[h(t)] \, dt \\ \int x_0(t)x[h(t)] \, dt & \int \{x[h(t)]\}^2 \, dt \end{array} \right] \qquad (7.5)$$

is singular, so only one of its eigenvalues is nonzero. This is also the case if we replace the integrals in the matrix by sums over a mesh of values t_j.

Consider, for example, the relation of the smooth variation in the temperature data to their periodic trend over 1989, shown in the left panel of Figure (7.8). Note the large loop in the lower left of this plot, due to the early arrival of winter in this year. The eigenvalues of the matrix (7.5) are 2.380 and 0.032. The smaller eigenvalue is positive because these two sets of curve values are not proportional to each other.

This line of reasoning suggests that we might choose the warping function $h(t)$ to minimize the logarithm of the smallest eigenvalue of the cross-product matrix (7.5). Denote this quantity by MINEIG(h). In cases like the printing data, where the functions are multivariate, we can form a composite criterion by adding the criterion across functions. The criterion often works even better if we use the first derivative values, or even a higher derivative if it can be estimated stably. This is because derivatives tend to oscillate more rapidly than functions, and also to vary about zero, so that the smallest eigenvalue measure is even more sensitive to whether functions differ only by amplitude variation.

We can see how these two techniques work on an artificial example. Let the target function be $x_0(t) = \sin 2\pi t$, and let the function to be registered be $x(t) = \sqrt{2}(\sin 2\pi t + \cos 2\pi t)$. These two functions have a phase difference of $1/8$, and $x(t)$ has a maximum of 2 as compared to the maximum of $x_0(t)$ of 1. Otherwise, the two functions have the same shape. The results are shown in the upper two panels of Figure 7.9, where we see that the registered function is a lateral shift by 0.125 of the unregistered function. In the upper-right panel, we see as expected that $h(t) \approx t$. The problem with the least squares criterion (7.3) can be seen in the bottom two panels. We see that this criterion is minimized in the presence of considerable amplitude differences by pinching in the larger curve over amplitudes where both the smaller and larger curve have values. The resulting warping function is far from diagonal, and even the lateral shift is poorly estimated, with a value of 0.117.

Returning to the registration of the temperature data, the right panel of Figure 7.8 shows that the registered smooth trend is more tightly related to a proportional relationship. The two eigenvalues are now 2.388 and 0.018, and, although the first eigenvalues hardly change at all, the second eigenvalue is now 57% of the corresponding value before registration.

A generalization, investigated by Kneip, Li, MacGibbon, and Ramsay (2000), is to replace the constant A by a smooth positive function $A_i(t)$ which does not vary too quickly. This allows local features of x_i to be

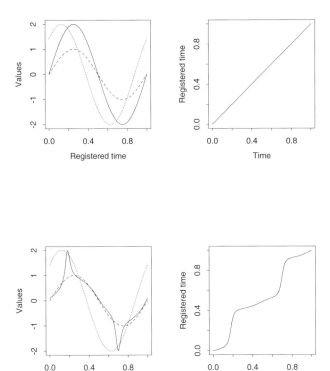

Figure 7.9. The upper two panels show results for an artificial registration problem using the minimum eigenvalue criterion. The dotted curve in the upper-left panel is the curve to be registered to the curve indicated by the dashed line. The solid line is the registered curve. The upper-right panel contains the warping function for this case, $h(t) = t$. The lower panels show the same results using the least squares criterion.

registered to those of x_0 even if the overall scale of variation is not constant across the whole range.

7.6.2   Estimation of the warping function

The software on the Web site associated with this chapter offers a choice between the two fitting criteria defined above: least squared error and minimum smallest eigenvalue of the cross-product matrix. Since the warping function $h(t)$ is strictly increasing, it can be represented using the methodology of Chapter 6 in terms of its relative acceleration $w(t) = h''(t)/h'(t)$. We can then permit a roughness penalty based on the mth derivative of $w(t)$, by minimizing

$$\text{MINEIG}_\lambda(h) = \text{MINEIG}(h) + \lambda \int \{w^{(m)}(t)\}^2 \, dt, \qquad (7.6)$$

or the corresponding criterion based on FSSE. In the analyses we have presented, the MINEIG criterion was used. For either criterion, if $m = 0$, larger values of the smoothing parameter λ shrink the relative acceleration w to zero, and therefore shrink $h(t)$ to t. In practice, it is satisfactory to choose the smoothing parameter λ subjectively.

If we need to estimate derivatives of $h(t)$, it may be better to work with higher values of m. This can happen, for example, if we want to use derivatives of the registered functions with respect to t, in which case the chain rule will require the corresponding derivatives of $h(t)$.

Our software represents the function w in terms of a B-spline expansion. Ramsay and Li (1998) use order 1 (piecewise linear) B-splines for w since this permits the expression of h in a closed form and leads to relatively fast computation. Higher-order splines can be used at the expense of some numerical integration.

8

How Do Bone Shapes Indicate Arthritis?

8.1   Introduction

In this chapter we return to the analysis of the bone shape data discussed in Chapter 4. The *intercondylar notch*, the inside of the inverted U-shape shown in Figure 1.5, is considered important by medical specialists. The anterior cruciate ligament runs through the intercondylar notch, and damage to this ligament is known to be a risk factor for osteoarthritis of the knee. Although other studies have examined large-scale features of the intercondylar notch, there has not been very much examination of its detailed shape, nor of its direct relationship to the incidence of osteoarthritis.

In Chapter 4 we studied the shape of the bone outline by considering a number of landmarks and interpolating between them. In this chapter we look much more closely at the shape of the intercondylar notch, by taking a more subtle approach to the detailed representation of the shapes.

We consider a set of 96 notch outlines, on each of which we have some concomitant information, such as the age of the individual and whether there is evidence of arthritic bone change. Our concentration on the notch alone allows us to include a number of partly damaged bones that could not be considered in Chapter 4; as long as any damage does not affect the notch it is no longer a problem. In the sample we consider there are 21 femora from arthritic individuals and 75 from individuals showing no signs of arthritic bone change. We use the data to demonstrate three aspects of functional data analysis.

Table 8.1. The coordinates of the lateral and medial edges of the intercondylar notch for one particular femur. The values Y give the pixel rows, numbered from top to bottom of the image. The values X_L and X_M give the lateral and medial positions within row Y of the edges of the intercondylar notch.

Y	X_L	X_M	Y	X_L	X_M	Y	X_L	X_M	Y	X_L	X_M
80	59	61	92	49	83	104	45	87	116	41	85
81	54	61	93	48	84	105	45	87	117	40	85
82	52	63	94	48	85	106	45	87	118	40	85
83	52	64	95	48	86	107	45	86	119	39	86
84	52	66	96	47	87	108	44	86	120	37	87
85	52	68	97	47	87	109	44	86	121	36	87
86	52	73	98	47	87	110	43	86	122	35	88
87	51	77	99	46	87	111	43	86	123	35	89
88	51	78	100	46	87	112	44	86	124	33	90
89	51	79	101	46	87	113	43	86	125	30	91
90	50	80	102	46	87	114	42	86	—	—	—
91	49	82	103	46	87	115	41	86	—	—	—

1. How do we handle curves and shapes without making use of landmarks?

2. What does principal components analysis tell us about the variability of these data?

3. What are the issues involved in developing a functional analogue of discriminant analysis?

Part of the object of the study is to understand the way in which arthritic and nonarthritic bones differ. We have information on this aspect in that some bones display eburnation, which is a consequence of arthritis. In this chapter we take eburnation to be synonymous with arthritis, but it could well be that some of the noneburnated bones are from individuals with arthritis that is mild or in its early stages. This means that any conclusions we reach about the differences between arthritic and nonarthritic bones are conservative.

8.2 Analyzing shapes without landmarks

The bone shapes are stored as 128×128 pixel images, obtained by processing pictures such as that in Figure 1.5. The pixels are numbered from the top to the bottom of the picture in the vertical direction, and from the lateral to the medial (the outside to the inside) in the horizontal direction. To record the shape of the notch, we move row by row up the pixel image, starting with the first row of pixels that touches the notch, and for each

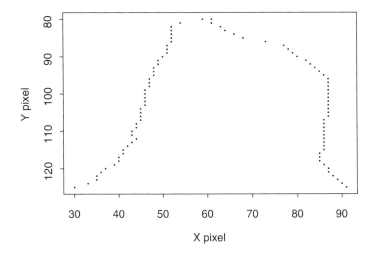

Figure 8.1. The raw data for the intercondylar notch for a particular individual. The lateral side is on the left and the medial on the right.

row find the pixel positions at either side of the notch. A specific example is given in Table 8.1 and plotted in Figure 8.1.

It can be seen from the figure that Y cannot be written as a simple function of X. For instance, as we move down the notch on the medial side, we first move out to pixel 87, then back to 85, and finally out to 91 again. Furthermore, a large part of this edge is vertical or nearly so. Merely considering Y as a function of X will not work; instead we will have to find a better way of parameterizing the shape of the notch.

A fruitful approach is *parameterization by arc length*. We define functions $x(t)$ and $y(t)$ such that as t increases from 0 to 1 the point $\{x(t), y(t)\}$ moves at a constant speed along the curve. We then regard the two-dimensional function $\mathbf{z}(t) = \{x(t), y(t)\}$ as being our functional datum. Landmarks are not required; instead the distance along the curve is used to yield the points whose coordinates are used for the subsequent analysis. Distance measured along a curve is called *arc length*.

To apply this approach to the data given in Table 8.1, first we connect the dots to obtain a continuous outline, as shown in Figure 8.2. In this figure, there is some rapid variation in the part of the curve on the lateral side, partly due to the pixelation of the image. We are not interested in variation on this scale. However, we wish to calculate distances along the curve in order to define the functions $x(t)$ and $y(t)$, and small scale variations will increase such arc lengths in a spurious way. Therefore we perform some

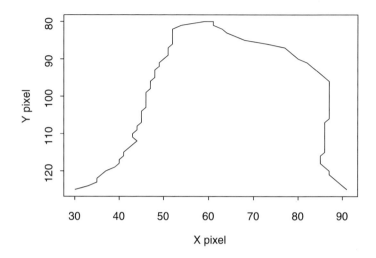

Figure 8.2. Joining the centers of the boundary pixels: the first step in producing a curve parameterized by arc length.

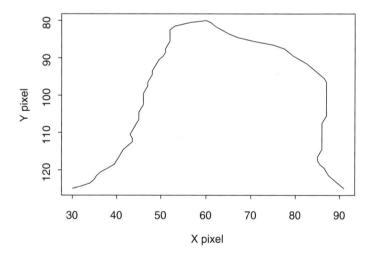

Figure 8.3. Smoothing by joining the midpoints of the line segments in Figure 8.2: the next step in producing a curve parameterized by arc length.

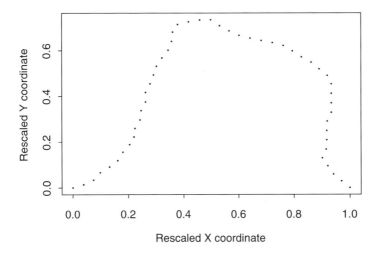

Figure 8.4. Fifty points equally spaced along the curve shown in Figure 8.3 with the curve rescaled to start and finish at standard positions. Interpolating these positions linearly is the final step in producing a curve parameterized by arc length.

very light smoothing, joining the midpoints between the dots, instead of the dots themselves. The effect, shown in Figure 8.3, is to reduce the local variability noticeably without changing the structure in any substantial way.

Only the shape of the notch is of interest, so we rescale the curve equally in both coordinate directions, and also shift it, to make it run from $(0,0)$ to $(1,0)$ in the X–Y plane. By calculating the distance along all the small line segments that make up Figure 8.3 we find 50 points (x_k, y_k) at equal arc length along the curve, as plotted in Figure 8.4. This process has yielded a fine grid of 50 points evenly spaced along the notch outline, capturing all the essential features of the shape of the intercondylar notch. Let $t_1 = 0, t_2 = 1/49, t_3 = 2/49, \ldots, t_{50} = 1$. To complete the specification of the shape as a curve parameterized by arc length, define the functions $x(t)$ and $y(t)$ by setting $x(t_k) = x_k$ and $y(t_k) = y_k$ for each k, and interpolating linearly between these points.

This process is applied to each of the $N = 96$ outlines in the sample. For each $j = 1, 2, \ldots, N$ we obtain a pair of functions $\{X_j(t), Y_j(t)\}$, written as the vector function $\mathbf{Z}_j(t)$. Each X_j and Y_j is held in discretized form, so the actual data are held in an $N \times 50 \times 2$ array, recording the coordinates of the 50 points picked out along each curve. The $(j, k, 1)$ element of this array is the X-coordinate of the kth point on the jth curve, and the $(j, k, 2)$ element the corresponding Y-coordinate. The choice of the number 50 is somewhat arbitrary, and our analyses are not particularly sensitive to this choice; because of the original pixelation of the data there is no point in trying to recover information on any smaller scale.

8.3   Investigating shape variation

8.3.1   Looking at means alone

We can define the notion of a mean shape, by finding the functions

$$\bar{X}(t) = N^{-1} \sum_i X_i(t) \quad \text{and} \quad \bar{Y}(t) = N^{-1} \sum_i Y_i(t),$$

and letting the mean shape be the curve traced out by the two-dimensional function $\bar{\mathbf{Z}}(t) = \{\bar{X}(t), \bar{Y}(t)\}$. In practice, we average over the first dimension of the data array to yield a 50×2 matrix giving the coordinates of 50 points along the mean curve; joining these points gives the mean curve $\bar{\mathbf{Z}}(t)$ plotted in Figure 8.5. The halfway point along this curve, for instance, is the average of all the halfway points on the individual curves.[1]

The means of the eburnated and noneburnated groups are plotted in Figure 8.6. It might appear that the distinguishing feature of the arthritic bones is that they have a shallower notch, because this is the way that the mean shapes differ. However, we show that a more careful statistical analysis does not yield the same conclusion, and that the mode of variability that best distinguishes the two groups is quite different.

8.3.2   Principal components analysis

Before considering further the subdivision into arthritic and nonarthritic bones, we investigate the ways in which the data set as a whole varies. Regarding the two-dimensional functions $\mathbf{Z}_i(t)$ as our functional data, functional PCA yields an expansion in terms of two-dimensional functions $\boldsymbol{\xi}_j(t) = \{\xi_j^X(t), \xi_j^Y(t)\}$. There are coefficients z_{ij} such that the observations can be expanded as

$$\mathbf{Z}_i(t) = \sum_{j \geq 1} z_{ij} \boldsymbol{\xi}_j(t). \tag{8.1}$$

---

[1]There is an interesting wrinkle here that is not relevant to our particular application: the points along the mean curve need not actually be themselves equally spaced, and in some cases it may be a good idea to go back and reparameterize the individual curves by reference to the way that the mean curve turns out. In our case this is not a problem.

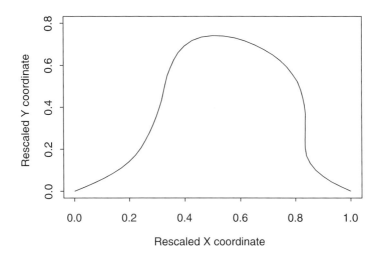

Figure 8.5. The mean notch shape curve.

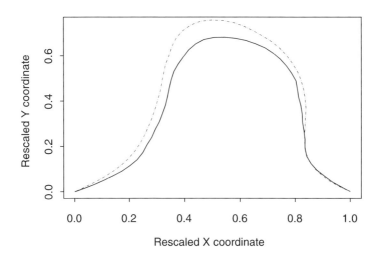

Figure 8.6. Solid: the mean curve for arthritic bones; dashed: the mean curve for nonarthritic bones.

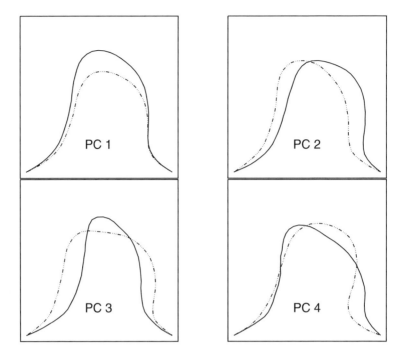

Figure 8.7. The first four principal components of variability of the notch shapes. The solid curves are the outlines corresponding to adding a multiple of the relevant weight function to the mean, and the dashed curves those obtained by subtracting the same multiple. The percentages of variability explained by these components are, respectively, 72.5, 13.9, 5.9, and 3.9%.

The actual PCA is performed by carrying out a standard PCA of the 100-vectors giving the coordinates of the points along the curves. It turns out that no smoothing is necessary.

To understand the principal component weight functions $\boldsymbol{\xi}_j(t)$, we can, as usual, plot $\overline{\mathbf{Z}}(t) \pm c\boldsymbol{\xi}_j(t)$ for some suitable multiple c. In this case the perturbed functions $\overline{\mathbf{Z}}(t) \pm c\boldsymbol{\xi}_j(t)$ are two-dimensional functions, and we plot their path in X–Y space as t varies. In Figure 8.7 the effects of the first four principal components of variability are displayed. These components together explain 96% of the variability in the data, with no other component explaining more than about 1% of the variability.

The displayed components all have simple interpretations. The first component corresponds to the depth of the notch, and the second to the shift of the notch relative to the bottom points of the condyles. The third component gives information about the width of the notch, and the fourth shows how convex the medial part of the notch tends to be.

The depth of the notch accounts for a great deal of the variability in the sample, and so in plotting Figure 8.7 the size of the perturbation shown in each part of the plot is not chosen by reference to the amount of variability in the original sample. Instead, the same multiple c of the principal component curve is used in each case, the multiple being chosen to make the mode of variability clear without grossly exaggerating it. Further details are given in the Web page associated with this chapter.

Thus far, the use of functional PCA for functions parameterized by arc length has no particular relation to the concomitant information that some of the bones are arthritic and some are not. In order to explore this aspect, we consider a different functional data analysis method, an extension of discriminant analysis. Apart from the way in which it identifies particular modes of variability within the population, the principal components analysis provides a convenient basis for the expression of the shapes in the sample and of other notch shapes.

8.4 The shape of arthritic bones

8.4.1 Linear discriminant analysis

Suppose that δ_i is a sequence of numbers such that $\delta_i = 1$ if the ith bone is arthritic and -1 if it is not. In the present context, the object of functional discriminant analysis is to find a vector function $\boldsymbol{\alpha}(t) = (\alpha_X(t), \alpha_Y(t))$ such that we can predict δ for any given bone (drawn either from the sample or from a new set of data) by calculating the discriminant values

$$\hat{\delta}_i = \int_0^1 \{X_i(t)\alpha_X(t)dt + Y_i(t)\alpha_Y(t)\}dt, \qquad (8.2)$$

and checking whether it lies above or below some critical value C.

The function $\boldsymbol{\alpha}(t)$ characterizes the mode of variability that best discriminates between the two populations. Moving away from the mean in the direction of $\boldsymbol{\alpha}(t)$ is the way of increasing the integral in (8.2) as fast as possible. But how is $\boldsymbol{\alpha}$ to be found?

Suppose the data were vectors Z_i rather than functions $\mathbf{Z}_i(t)$. The corresponding problem would be to find a vector a and a constant C such that we could predict the population from which a vector Z was drawn by calculating whether $a'Z > C$. The classical method called *linear discriminant analysis* finds the vector a that minimizes the ratio of the within-group sum of squares to the between-group sum of squares. Let $\bar{Z}^{(1)}$ and $\bar{Z}^{(2)}$ be the means of the two populations and let $\hat{S}$ be the pooled estimate of the variance matrix. Then the linear discriminant method yields

$$a = \hat{S}^{-1}(\bar{Z}^{(2)} - \bar{Z}^{(1)})$$

and

$$C = \tfrac{1}{2}a'(\bar{Z}^{(2)} + \bar{Z}^{(1)}).$$

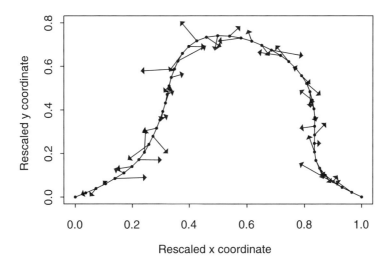

Figure 8.8. The mode of variability corresponding to a linear discriminant analysis carried out directly on the matrix of coordinates defining the notch shapes. The arrows show how the 50 defining points on the mean curve are perturbed in the direction defined by the discriminant vector. The way to increase the discriminant score most quickly is to move away from the mean shape in the direction of the arrows.

In the functional case, we have observations on 100 variables, the X- and Y-coordinates of the points around the notch, for each of the N individuals in the sample. Naively, we could apply the linear discriminant method to these high-dimensional vectors. The resulting 100-vector a can be translated back into a 50×2 matrix of weights corresponding to a mode of variability in the space of possible notch shapes.

Unfortunately this approach does not give a meaningful result. See Figure 8.8 for the mode of variability that it yields. This mode of variability clearly cannot be associated with any genuine feature of the problem in hand. Furthermore, this discriminant has the property that it classifies every bone in the sample perfectly; every arthritic bone has $a'Z > C$ and every nonarthritic bone has $a'Z < C$. However superficially attractive such performance may be, it is scarcely credible as a result of the study.

This phenomenon—gross overfitting combined with an apparently meaningless discriminant function—is an intrinsic feature of the naive approach, and has nothing to do with the arthritis data in particular. It has a mathematical explanation touched upon in Chapter 12 of Ramsay and Silverman

(1997) and discussed in more detail in references given there. In the present context a more informal explanation is given in Section 8.6.2 below.

8.4.2   Regularizing the discriminant analysis

We have to apply some regularization in order to give meaningful answers. A simple method is to expand the data in terms of some suitable basis, and only to consider a finite number of terms in this basis, both in the expansion of the data themselves and in the specification of the discriminant weight function $(\alpha_X(t), \alpha_Y(t))$.

In the present case, the principal components analysis gives a low-dimensional representation of the data that preserves as much as possible of the sample variability. For this reason we use as our basis expansion the harmonics provided by the functional PCA of the data themselves. Fix some fairly small integer J and consider only the first J terms in the principal components expansion (8.1) of each of the functions. For concreteness we choose $J = 6$. For each bone, we then have six principal component scores on which to base our linear discriminant, and we apply standard discriminant analysis to the $N \times 6$ matrix $(z_{ij}, i = 1, \ldots, N; j = 1, \ldots, 6)$. This yields a vector a of length 6, giving a linear discriminant in terms of the principal component scores,

$$\hat{\delta}_i = \sum_{j=1}^{6} a_j z_{ij}. \tag{8.3}$$

We can express the discriminant value in terms of the notch curves themselves. By standard properties of principal component expansions,

$$z_{ij} = \int_0^1 \{X_i(t)\xi_j^X(t) + Y_i(t)\xi_j^Y(t)\}dt$$

for each i and j. Substituting into (8.3), the linear discriminant value $\hat{\delta}_i$ satisfies

$$\begin{aligned}
\hat{\delta}_i &= \sum_{j=1}^{6} a_j \int_0^1 \{X_i(t)\xi_j^X(t) + Y_i(t)\xi_j^Y(t)\}dt \\
&= \int_0^1 \{\alpha_X(t)X_i(t) + \alpha_Y(t)Y_i(t)\}dt,
\end{aligned}$$

where

$$\begin{bmatrix} \alpha_X(t) \\ \alpha_Y(t) \end{bmatrix} = \sum_{j=1}^{6} a_j \begin{bmatrix} \xi_j^X(t) \\ \xi_j^Y(t) \end{bmatrix}. \tag{8.4}$$

Comparing with equation (8.2), we can consider the two-dimensional function $\boldsymbol{\alpha}(t) = \{\alpha_X(t), \alpha_Y(t)\}$ as defining the functional linear discriminant between the two groups of bones.

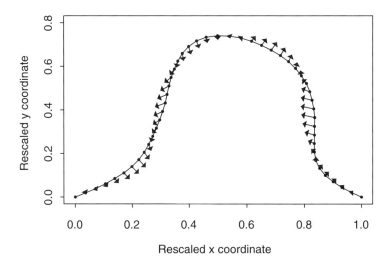

Figure 8.9. The mode of variability corresponding to a functional linear discriminant $\alpha(t)$ based on the first six principal components of the notch shape data. The solid curve is the mean shape, and the arrows show the direction in which the discriminant score increases most rapidly.

The mode of variability corresponding to the resulting $\alpha(t)$ is displayed in Figure 8.9. Bones with a higher discriminant score will have an intercondyle notch twisted to the left in the way that the figure is plotted. Because the mean is somewhat twisted to the right, this will tend to make the notch more symmetrical and to have a right edge that is less concave. The arthritic bones will tend to be in this category, and the average difference between the two groups of bones is approximately that corresponding to the lengths of the arrows in Figure 8.9.

The number J may be thought of as a *regularization parameter*, which determines how far we regularize the problem in order to produce our estimate. If we set J very small, equal to 1, for example, then the discrimination can only be based on a single principal component and important information may be lost. On the other hand, if J is chosen too large, then we will get the kind of spurious results discussed in Section 8.4.1 above. As in many smoothing and regularization contexts it is often sufficient to experiment with different values of the regularization parameter and choose between them by inspection, and in this case such inspection will immediately rule out values of J greater than about 12. However, it is also helpful to have criteria to help make this choice, and one of these is a cross-validation method described further in Section 8.6.3. This method confirms our choice $J = 6$.

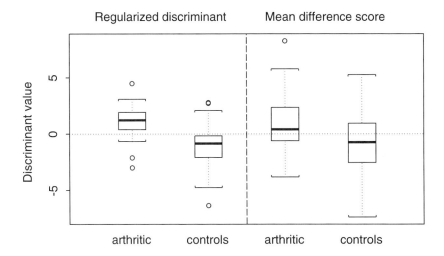

Figure 8.10. Box plots of discriminant scores. The two plots on the left give linear discriminant scores based on the first six principal components. Those on the right give scores based on the difference between the group means. The scores are scaled so that the arthritic bones have mean 1 and the nonarthritic mean -1. Note that the boxes in the first two plots do not overlap at all, whereas there is considerable overlap between the boxes in the last two plots. In every case the box covers the middle 50% of the relevant sample.

8.4.3 Why not just look at the group means?

The mode of variability that best discriminates between the arthritic and nonarthritic bones picks out features that are not at all apparent in the simple comparison of the means in Figure 8.6. Is this a contradiction?

The two curves in Figure 8.6 differ almost entirely along the lines of the first principal component of variability of the population as a whole, shown in Figure 8.7 to correspond to the depth of the notch. There is considerable population variation in this component, and hence in the notch depth, and this general variation is reflected in the differences in the mean notch depths for the two subpopulations. If we project all the data on the direction of the difference between the mean curves, the t-statistic for the difference between the two subpopulations is about 3.1.

On the other hand, if we consider the linear discriminant scores based on the first six principal components, the t-statistic for the difference between the two groups is 4.8. The regularized linear discriminant is much better at separating the two groups than is the direction of variability defined by the group means. Figure 8.10 gives a graphic presentation of this: the two scores are each rescaled so that the mean of the arthritic bones is $+1$ and the mean of the controls is -1. The box plots show that the "six principal component linear discriminant" approach separates the subpopulations far better than the "mean difference projection direction."

8.5   What have we seen?

The right way to express shapes in functional form may not always be obvious. If our object is a curve in two dimensions then parameterization by arc length can be a convenient way of representing the functional observations as vector-valued functions $\{x(t), y(t)\}$ of a scalar parameter t. Standard methods such as functional PCA can then be used to analyze the data. Without such a parameterization even the notion of a mean curve has no obvious definition.

Linear discriminant analysis can be extended to the functional context, but regularization is necessary to give meaningful results. Intuitively, if an entire function is used to predict a single quantity, such as the class to which the function belongs, then a totally spurious feature of the function may give perfect prediction for the particular data set observed. One possible regularization approach is to concentrate on the first few principal components, or some other finite-dimensional representation of the data. Whatever method of regularization is used, the regularization parameter can be chosen by inspection or by an approach like cross-validation.

Functional discriminant analysis can distinguish groups better than consideration of the group mean curves alone. The group means may differ in ways that reflect modes of variability in the population generally, rather than those that specifically separate the groups within the population. The means of the two subpopulations might suggest that it is the depth of the notch that is associated with the symptoms of arthritis. However, the functional discriminant analysis indicates that the best discriminating characteristic is the differing amout of "twist" in the notch shape. This aspect of the shape could affect the way that the anterior cruciate ligament lies in the intercondylar notch, with a possible link to arthritis as discussed in Section 8.1. Within the present study, we cannot disentangle the influence of bone shape on arthritis from the possibility that arthritis causes a change in bone shape. However, our results give clues and pointers for future work in the fields of rheumatology and biomechanics.

8.6   Notes and further issues

8.6.1   Bibliography

The notch shape study discussed is a reworking of Shepstone, Rogers, Kirwan, and Silverman (2001), which deals with the same data and the same clinical issues, but uses a somewhat different approach to the parameterization of the notch shapes and to the subsequent analysis. That paper contains full details of the medical background, including key references to work in the rheumatological, biomechanical, and veterinary literature.

Functional discriminant analysis is a particular example of the use of functions as predictors, as discussed broadly by Ramsay and Silverman (1997, Chapter 10). They treat in detail the general necessity for regularization in such problems, and consider various approaches to regularization, including roughness penalty methods. An early paper in the FDA literature dealing with these issues is Leurgans, Moyeed, and Silverman (1993), who demonstrate and investigate the need for regularization in another functional context, canonical correlation analysis. Hastie, Buja and Tibshirani (1995) set out the general idea of functional discriminant analysis making use of a roughness penalty approach to regularization. They apply their methods to a problem in speech recognition and to the classification of digits in handwritten postal addresses. Both functional canonical correlation analysis and functional discriminant analysis are treated in detail in Ramsay and Silverman (1997, Chapter 12).

8.6.2 Why is regularization necessary?

We can give an intuitive argument for the necessity of regularization for the bone shape discriminant problem. The discretized coordinates of the data provide N points in 100-dimensional space. Four of the coordinates are fixed, because the notches are all scaled to start at $(0, 1)$ and end at $(1, 1)$, so the points are essentially in 96-dimensional space. We set the elements of a corresponding to these four fixed coordinates to zero. Now consider any division of the points into two groups, red and blue, say, and suppose that we want to find a vector a such that $a'Z_i = 1$ if Z_i is a red point, and $a'Z_i = -1$ if Z_i is a blue point. These are N equations in the 96 unknowns in a, and so, because $N = 96$, there is a solution that gives perfect discrimination between the populations. If we had used a finer discretization of the notches then there would have been N equations in even more unknowns, and hence an infinite set of such solutions. To put it less precisely, there is so much freedom in the choice of the vector a that it is not surprising that some completely uninteresting direction happens to give a discriminant function that works excellently on the given data but is in fact spurious—of course it will not have any value for classifying any new data collected.

This intuitive argument points to the qualitative difference between the regularization of functional discriminant analysis and roughness penalty smoothing as applied to PCA (as discussed in Chapter 2). For discriminant analysis, regularization is a mathematical necessity, however well behaved the original data—indeed, for mathematical reasons we do not go into here, the smoother the data the more acute the need for regularization. On the other hand, for functional PCA, smoothing is only important when we have data of high intrinsic variability, as we did in Chapter 2; an unsmoothed analysis will often suffice.

8.6.3 Cross-validation in classification problems

The best approach to assessing the quality of a discriminant is to go out and collect completely new data and to see how well the discriminant rule based on the original data works on these new data. Unfortunately, in many contexts there are no new data available, and so we have to make use of the data we have. The simplest assessment of the discriminant is the *resubstitution* approach: feed the original data back through the discriminant, and see how well classified they are. This approach will usually be optimistic. The *leave-one-out cross-validation* method attempts to avoid the use of the same data both to train and to test the discriminant as follows: classify each data point using a discriminant constructed from all the data except that particular point. This requires a separate discriminant function for each data point in the sample and so may be computationally intensive, although there are some computational shortcuts that can be used. The approach is reminiscent of the cross-validation method when estimating the mean in the way described in Section 2.6.

Table 8.2. The cross-validation counts of false positives and false negatives for various values of the number J of principal components used in the discriminant algorithm. To get misclassification rates, divide the first row by 75 and the second row by 21.

J	1	2	3	4	5	6	7	8	9	10	11	12
False pos	26	27	22	22	23	19	23	21	21	22	22	22
False neg	10	8	8	8	8	7	7	7	7	7	8	9

Because the cross-validation approach gives a classification for each point individually, we can count both the number of false positives (nonarthritic bones that are classified as arthritic) and the number of false negatives (arthritic bones that fail to be so classified). The results are tabulated for various values of J in Table 8.2. In some circumstances we might need to combine false positive and false negative rates into a single score, but the choice $J = 6$ is the unique value that minimizes both scores, and so would be the minimum whatever linear combination of the two scores we were to choose.

A final comparison relevant to the discussion of Section 8.4.3 can be obtained by calculating the leave-one-out cross-validation scores for the approach of projecting on the difference between the two group means. This yields false positive and negative rates of 25 and 9, respectively, noticeably worse than the values of 19 and 7 yielded by the discriminant based on the first six principal components.

9
Functional Models for Test Items

9.1 Introduction

After our bank accounts and our taxes, it is hard to imagine data playing a more central role in our lives than the examinations, opinion surveys, attitude questionnaires, and psychological scales administered to ourselves, our children, and our students. These data may not on first impression appear to be functional, but we show that functional data analysis can reveal how both test takers and test items perform in test situations. To provide a concrete frame of reference, we look at the responses of 5000 examinees to 60 items in a test of mathematics achievement developed by the American College Testing Program. We apply functional principal components analysis to explore variation across test items, and we check the fairness of certain items by comparing male and female performance. Finally, we use a functional property of these data to develop a useful new way of describing the performance of individual examinees.

Let us assume that each of n items is given to each of N examinees, and that each item is answered either correctly or incorrectly. We record each response with a value of 1 if examinee j answers item i correctly, and 0 otherwise. We want to use these data, crude as they may seem, to provide a reasonable answer to the question, "What is the probability P_{ij} that examinee j gets item i right?"

Since we have only a single 0/1 datum to estimate P_{ij}, we obviously need to make some simplifying assumptions. We can take advantage of the fact that exam performances are not really all that unique; given this many examinees, an arbitrary examinee j is likely to have lots of "neighbors" in the sense of other examinees who get about the same number of right and wrong answers. Moreover, we will likely see that they even distribute these answers in a roughly similar manner. To a first approximation, poorly performing examinees will tend to get only the same easy items right, and strong examinees will fail only the same small subset of extremely hard items. Thus, we can pool information across similar examinees if we can propose a reasonable way of defining "similar."

9.2   The ability space curve

Figure 9.1 captures an idea that underlies almost all models for test data. We have plotted estimates of these right answer probabilities P_{ij} for three test items on the ACT exam. Using a techique outlined below, these probabilities were estimated for 21 prototypical examinees, selected across the whole range of ability. Note that these are not actual candidates; rather, the observed data are used to obtain estimates of the probabilities of success for various items as the ability of the candidate varies in some way. Items 1, 9, and 59 were selected for Figure 9.1 because they are, respectively, low, medium, and high in difficulty. We can see that most of the 21 examinee points are high along the Item 1 axis, indicating that Item 1 is easy. Item 59's difficulty is demonstrated by the fact that most points are low along the corresponding axis, and because many points are in the middle of the range on the Item 9 axis, that item is somewhere between these two in difficulty.

The points corresponding to examinees fall along a curve. At the near end in Figure 9.1 are the poor students who pass all three items with probabilities near 0, and at the far end are those who rejoice in near certainty of passing all three. We use the term *space curve* to refer to a curve like this in a space of three or more dimensions. Of course, Figure 9.1 is only an incomplete picture; what we really have in mind is the space curve within 60-dimensional space, the coordinates of which are the probabilities of success on each of the 60 items. The *smoothness* of this space curve, or its continuum character, reflects a belief that probabilities of success will change smoothly as we change ability. Now of course there is such a thing as sudden insight, but the data collected by large testing agencies administering examinations to millions of people a year supports this assumption of a steady change in probability, at least for answers to multiple choice exam questions and for most examinees.

Our usual practice of summarizing test performance by a single score, such as number correct, also reflects these notions of unidimensionality and smoothness. We consider examinees as tending to vary in essentially one way that we refer to as low-to-high ability. When we group together ex-

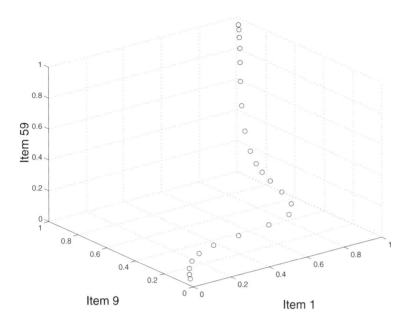

Figure 9.1. Each circle plots the three probabilities of success on items 1, 9, and 56 in the ACT math test for an examinee. The nearest 3 points are for examinees likely to fail all three items, and the far 3 points are examinees likely to succeed on all three. These 21 points fall along a smooth space curve within the unit cube.

aminees with the same test score, we expect to find that their patterns of right and wrong answers are not all that different. We also find that, as we move between nearby scores, the changes in these patterns are comparatively small. Indeed, tests are designed this way, by selecting items we know in advance will be easy, average, or hard. In short, if you are an average student taking a well-designed test, you and most other average students will fail the hard items, get the easy ones right, and differ from each other mostly in terms of the items that match your ability.

Thus, a plausible way to define "similar" for pairs of examinees is in terms of small differences in test scores. Two examinees have performances in the same "neighborhood" if their test scores are close together. We refine this notion later, but this seems like a reasonable place to start.

Any space curve can be defined by letting the coordinates of points on the curve be functions of a single variable. Consider, for example, a set of points in 3-D with coordinate values X_i, Y_i, and Z_i, and let these coordinate values be defined in terms of variable z by the equations

$$
\begin{aligned}
X_i &= \sin(\pi z_i) \\
Y_i &= \cos(\pi z_i) \\
Z_i &= z_i.
\end{aligned}
\tag{9.1}
$$

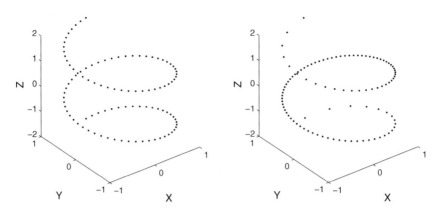

Figure 9.2. The locations of the points on the spiral in the left panel are determined by equations (9.1) for 101 equally-spaced values of z between -2 and 2. In the right panel the points are determined by values of z having a normal distribution.

Then the left panel of Figure 9.2 shows what happens if we let the variable z_i take on 101 equally spaced values between -2 and 2. The variable z is called the *charting variable*.

What if we made the values of z have values at equal percentage points of a normal distribution within these limits? The result is in the right panel of Figure 9.2. Although the spacings between points have changed, the shape of the spiral has not. From this example, we can infer that the shape of a space curve will not change if we make any smooth order-preserving transformation of the variable z. This principle explains why we can have many different mapping systems for charting out the surface of the earth; the earth is the same whichever we use, but particular choices are more convenient for some purposes than others.

Let us therefore define examinee j's position on the test performance curve in Figure 9.1 by the value θ_j of some charting variable θ. Then what Figure 9.1 displays, and what is redisplayed in Figure 9.3, are the functions $P_i(\theta)$ indicating how probability of success on item i varies over values of variable θ. It seems reasonable to call θ a measure in some sense of "ability" or "proficiency," and it is referred to by psychologists as the *latent trait* underlying performance on the exam. The functions $P_i(\theta)$ are called *item response functions* or *item characteristic curves*.

However, our spiral example shows us that there is no unique way to define the variable θ that maps out the space curve. Psychometricians usually resolve this ambiguity by fiat by imposing the restriction that the values of θ in the population of examinees have a standard normal distribution, along the lines of the right panel of Figure 9.2. This choice is arbitrary, but it does reflect the long-standing assumption, or perhaps tradition, that

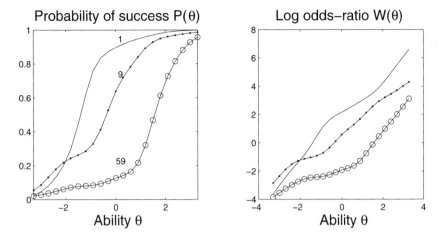

Figure 9.3. The three items displayed in Figure 9.1 are plotted in the left panel as functions $P_i(\theta)$ of the latent variable θ. The right panel contains the plots of the corresponding log odds-ratio functions $W_i(\theta)$

ability has a roughly normal distribution. The classic example is IQ as a measure of intellectual ability. We will return to this issue later and propose an alternative variable that has some useful properties.

9.3   Estimating item response functions

Probability functions such as $P_i(\theta)$ present special computational challenges because they are constrained to take values only between 0 and 1. We can deal with this constraint by applying a suitable transformation, and a convenient reformulation of $P_i(\theta)$ is

$$P_i(\theta) = \frac{\exp[W_i(\theta)]}{1 + \exp[W_i(\theta)]} \;, \qquad W_i(\theta) = \log \frac{P_i(\theta)}{1 - P_i(\theta)} \;. \tag{9.2}$$

Values of $W_i(\theta)$ near 0 correspond to success probabilities in the vicinity of 0.5, large negative Ws to very low Ps, and large positive Ws to near certainty of success. The function $W_i(\theta)$ is called the *log odds-ratio* function, and there are no constraints on its value.

The simple linear model

$$W_i(\theta) = a_i(\theta - b_i) \tag{9.3}$$

is one of the standard parametric models in psychometric theory, the two-parameter logistic model, or *2PL model* among those in the trade. Parameter b_i of this model is called the *difficulty* of the item and captures the location of the log odds-ratio function, by specifying the value for which $P_i(\theta) = \frac{1}{2}$. The slope parameter a_i is called the *discriminability* of the item, and is an index of how well the test item distinguishes between test takers as θ varies. Although the curves $W_i(\theta)$ that we estimate for this test will usually be more complex in shape than this, these two qualities of location and slope are fundamental descriptors of item performance.

In practice, the 2PL model is too simple because for most multiple choice tests even the weakest examinees can achieve a positive success rate merely by guessing. Consequently, the industry standard model is the three-parameter logistic model or *3PL model*, which uses an additional parameter c_i indicating this low-ability success probability, and has the structure,

$$P_i(\theta) = c_i + (1 - c_i)\frac{\exp[a_i(\theta - b_i)]}{1 + \exp[a_i(\theta - b_i)]} \; . \tag{9.4}$$

See Lord (1980) for a review of modern test theory and a wide range of applications of this model.

How do we estimate these log-odds functions $W_i(\theta)$ for each item, not knowing in advance what the independent variable values θ_j are for each examinee? The EM algorithm (Dempster, Laird, and Rubin, 1977) is used, in which θ_j is treated as if it were a missing datum. The EM algorithm proceeds by alternating between a phase called the E-step in which the item response functions are assumed known and likelihood is averaged over possible values of θ, and the M-step in which the θ_js are assumed available for a small number of prototypical examinees and the functions $W_i(\theta)$ are estimated.

We achieved much more flexibility than in (9.3) or in (9.4) by expanding $W_i(\theta)$ in terms of 11 B-spline basis functions using equally spaced knots. We used a penalized EM algorithm, which maximizes the likelihood but also imposes a certain amount of smoothness on these estimated functions by using a roughness penalty based on the log odds-ratio. Details are found in Rossi, Wang, and Ramsay (2002).

9.4   PCA of log odds-ratio functions

Let us assume that the item response functions $P_i(\theta)$ and their log-odds equivalents $W_i(\theta)$ have been estimated to our satisfaction. We now want to explore how these functions vary from item to item.

Functional principal components analysis can reveal interesting aspects of the variation among these items. Because they are unconstrained, we apply PCA to the log odds-ratio functions instead of the probability functions. In this section we focus attention on functions estimated from the 2115 male candidates. The first four principal components of the 60 log odds-ratio functions then account for 96% of the variation; although there are quite a large number of test items, their characteristics are captured essentially completely by variability in four dimensions. Figure 9.4 shows

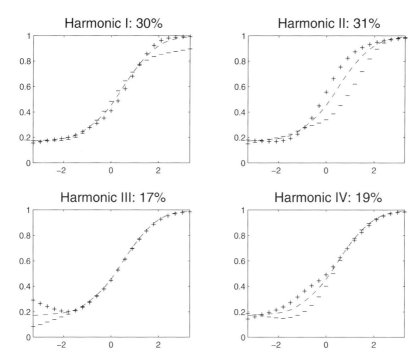

Figure 9.4. Each panel displays a varimax-rotated principal component of the variation among the log odds-ratio functions $W_i(\theta)$ estimated for the male candidates. A small multiple of each component is added (+) and subtracted (-) from the mean function, and the results transformed to probability functions, along the mean function. The percentages indicate percentages of variance accounted for, the total of which is 96%.

these four principal components after a varimax rotation to aid interpretation. These rotated components are displayed by adding and subtracting a small multiple of each component to the mean function $\bar{W}(\theta)$, and then back-transforming these perturbed means to their probability counterparts using (9.2).

These components can now be interpreted. Components I and III account for variation in characteristics of test items in the high and low ability ranges, respectively; components II and IV concentrate on variation over larger parts of the ability range, higher for component II and lower for component IV. An item with a high score on component I will be particularly good at sorting out very high ability students from others of moderately high ability, whereas if its score is low it will discriminate well among most of the population but will be found approximately of equal difficulty by all the very good students. Even the best students will not be certain of getting the item correct, a type of variation that the industry-standard 3PL model is unable to capture. However, we would be wise to

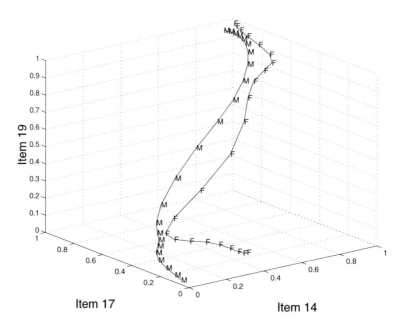

Figure 9.5. The space curves for items 14, 17, and 19 for men (M) and women (F).

remind ourselves that, even though the original data set is large, variation in the log-odds functions for extreme θ values is necessarily estimated by relatively small numbers of examinees, so conclusions for the extremes of the ability range should be treated with some caution.

An item with a high score on Component II would have a higher slope near the middle of the ability range and a lower slope for candidates with θ values approaching 2. Such an item gains local discriminability for average candidates at the expense of discriminability for the more able students. Similarly, Component IV quantifies a discriminability trade-off between average candidates and those with rather low abilities.

9.5   Do women and men perform differently on this test?

The ACT math test was taken by 2885 women and 2115 men. Figure 9.5 shows the space curves plotted in Figure 9.1 for both men and women for three different items. We see that performance on these three items evolves differently, and we may wish to investigate if there is something unusual about these three items.

We need a gold-standard summary of performance on the test such that for men and women having the same level on this summary, we can consider that they are roughly equivalent in ability. We cannot use θ for this purpose, since we have forced this parameter to have a standard normal distribution within each group. In particular, the mean θ value is zero for each group, regardless of any way that the groups might differ in overall performance. The reason that the comparison is difficult is that there may be differences in the pattern of performance, not merely its level. What we need is a way of comparing the separately estimated θ values for women with θ values for men.

The performance measure that comes to mind immediately is the number of right answers as a function of θ, and the expected value of this is

$$\tau(\theta) = \sum_i^n P_i(\theta) \ .$$

This *expected score* $\tau(\theta)$ measure of performance is often used by psychometricians to compare people in different groups.

However, we can propose some modifications of this idea. First, we might use the expected log odds-ratio, since in general it is wiser to take averages of unconstrained functions for the same reasons that we preferred to use PCA on the log odds-ratios. Once computed, we can back-transform this mean to the probability scale, and multiply it by the number of items to get what we might call a *fair score*. Second, we compute the expected value only using those items that do not appear to have gender differences in performance, so as to not contaminate our measure. In fact, only the three items plotted in Figure 9.5 appear to show much gender separation, so we use

$$\overline{W}(\theta) = (n-3)^{-1} \sum_{i \neq 14,17,19}^n W_i(\theta) \ ,$$

which we then back-transform to get our fair score

$$\tau(\theta) = \frac{\exp[\overline{W}(\theta)]}{1 + \exp[\overline{W}(\theta)]},$$

which we estimate separately for men and for women.

Figure 9.6 plots probabilities of success against fair score for men and women on items 17 and 19. Item 17 seems to favor men over most of the fair score range, and item 19 favors women. Item 14 is not plotted, but also favors men. These items exhibit what psychometricians call *differential item functioning*, abbreviated DIF. In the present context, it would probably make most sense in future tests to discard these three items altogether. An interesting question of a nonstatistical nature is to ask what is it that makes these mathematical items easier for one gender than another, when most are gender-neutral. It is especially interesting that the difference is not all in one direction.

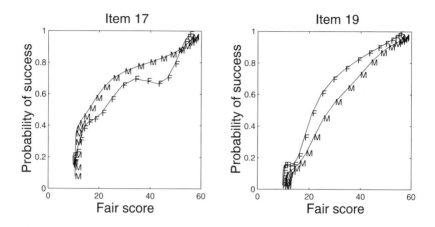

Figure 9.6. Probabilities of success for items 17 and 19 are plotted against a fair score that is a reasonable basis for equating ability of men and women.

9.6   A nonlatent trait: Arc length

In principle, there is nothing wrong with choosing the charting variable θ the way psychometricians do; the choice is arbitrary, and if one likes to think of ability as normally distributed, their choice is appealing. Unfortunately, users of test theory models, and some psychometricians as well, have tended to lose sight of the arbitrariness of the choice, and fall into thinking that the values θ_j measure ability in the same metric sense that the marks on a ruler measure length. It has been claimed, in fact, that this is one of the big arguments for using latent trait theory to model test performance.

Actually, there is a charting variable that really does have the metric properties that users and theorists would like to see, and is moreover not at all latent. This is *arc length*, s, the distance along the space curve determined by the simultaneous changes in probability as we move along the curve. We have already used arc length to advantage in Chapter 8 as a way of describing curves in two dimensions.

Arc length resists misinterpretation because small changes Δs in distance along the curve really do have a meaning that does depend on our present position. Distances along the curve are directly related to the changes in probabilities of success for the test items. Like units of physical measurement, arc length differences can meaningfully be added and subtracted.

The values of arc length s are computed by beginning with some arbitrary charting variable such as θ, estimating the corresponding item response functions $P_i(\theta)$ and their derivatives $P_i'(\theta)$, and then computing arc length

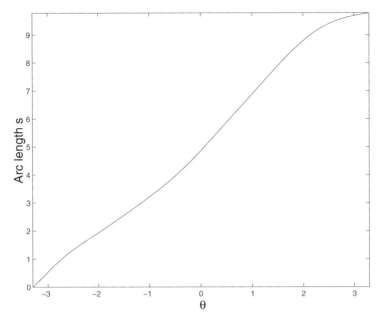

Figure 9.7. Arc length from a reference point, or the distance along the ability space curve, as a function of standard normal latent variable θ.

$s(\theta)$ by the equation

$$s(\theta) = \int_{\theta_0}^{\theta} \left\{ \sum_i [P_i'(u)]^2 \right\}^{1/2} du. \tag{9.5}$$

In this equation θ_0 is the lowest value of θ on the curve.

Arc length is called the *intrinsic metric* of the space curve, because its values do not depend on what kind of charting variable we use in (9.5). For the spiral in Figure 9.2, the 101 equally spaced values between 0 and $4\sqrt{2}$ are of equal arc distance along the curve.

For the male candidates in the math test, with the usual charting variable θ having a standard normal distribution, arc length $s(\theta)$ is displayed as a function of θ in Figure 9.7. We see that, in fact, the relationship is close to linear for all except the highest values of θ. Therefore, in this context arc length does not represent any dramatic departure from the traditional θ measure. The reference point from which arc length is measured corresponds to the performance of the weakest examinee.

For purposes of communicating with a user community, we would not mislead anyone much by linearly rescaling arc length to have an upper limit of 100 while retaining the lower limit of 0. The metric properties of this rescaled measure would still hold. Alternatively, as the Educational Testing Service and other large testing agencies do, we can pick lower and upper

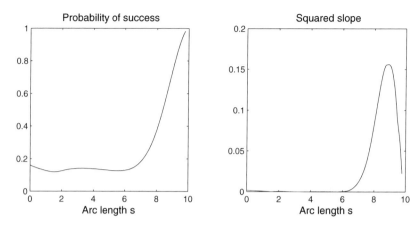

Figure 9.8. The left panel contains the item response function for item 56 as a function of arc length s, and the right panel contains its squared slope, a normalized measure of item quality. Only items 57 and 60 are this discriminating for high performance examinees.

fixed limits and rescale arc length to be within these limits. This would still be a metric measure of performance in the sense that differences can be added.

The elements $P_i'(s)$ of the tangent vector are the slopes of the item response functions at arc length s, and therefore measure the discriminability of the item. Arc length as a charting value has a useful property for assessing the quality of an item. Because we move at a steady speed along the curve as arc distance increases, the length of the tangent vector $\{P_1'(s), \ldots, P_n'(s)\}$ is exactly 1 when the curve is parameterized by arc length. Thus,

$$\sum_{i=1}^{n} \left(\frac{dP_i}{ds} \right)^2 = 1.$$

Since the squares of the discriminability estimates must sum to one, we can compare them across items by plotting $[P_i'(s)]^2$. The test items particularly contributing to discriminability will be different at different parts of the ability range.

For example, test developers find it hard to construct an item that discriminates well for examinees at the upper end of the ability continuum. Item 56 turns out to be such an item, and Figure 9.8 displays its item response function and its squared slope or discriminability as functions of arc length. The fact that the latter exceeds 0.15 and that the sum across all items of squared discriminability is 1 means that few items are this discriminating. In fact, only this and items 57 and 60 achieve any quality for high-end examinees.

We have highlighted items 56, 57, and 60 by considering the components of the tangent vector as functions of arc length. These results can be related to the principal components analysis carried out above. The four lowest principal scores for Component II are for items 56, 57, 59, and 60. The items also have large negative scores on Component IV. Figure 9.4 and the discussion of the components in Section 9.4 indicate that items with negative scores on both these components will be best at sorting out able students from one another.

9.7   What have we seen?

Functional data analysis is not only a method for analyzing observed curves; it can also be applied to curves implied by and estimated from data that are not at all curvaceous at first sight. Any single test datum does not by itself provide a lot of information about the item success probability P_{ij}, but by making the strong simplifying assumption that these probabilities vary in a smooth one-dimensional way across examinees, we can estimate the ability space curve that this assumption implies.

Once we have chosen a charting variable θ to measure out positions along this space curve, we can also study the n item response functions $P_i(\theta)$ as if they were a sample of observed functions. Actually, though, we are perhaps better off applying functional data analysis to the log odds-ratio functions $W_i(\theta)$, since these transformations of the item response functions have the unconstrained variation that we are used to seeing in directly observed curves. Principal components analysis seems like the ideal tool to study variations among these curves, and we found that the dimensionality of this variation was perhaps surprisingly small, and quite interpretable.

In the test item context, arc length is an attractive method of parameterizing ability. Arc length is not latent, may be less confusing to the practitioners of psychometrics, and offers an interesting new way of assessing item quality by plotting the square of the test discriminability function.

9.8   Notes and bibliography

To read more about modern test theory and its applications using parametric models, see Lord (1980) and the more classic Lord and Novick (1968). The EM algorithm was first applied to the estimation of parametric models in test theory by Bock and Aitkin (1981). Our use of the EM algorithm to estimate the functions $P_i(\theta)$ and $W_i(\theta)$ nonparametrically is based on theses by Wang (1993) and Rossi (2001), and are described in Rossi, Wang, and Ramsay (2002). The use of ideas from differential geometry to present nonparametric modern test theory comes from Ramsay (1995) and (1996a).

10

Predicting Lip Acceleration from Electromyography

10.1 The neural control of speech

Physiologists and psychologists who study motor control aim to understand how the brain controls movement. We know that waves of neural activation cascade down complex neural pathways to the motoneurons that activate muscle tissue, and that the contraction of these muscles applies forces to limbs. We know, too, from elementary physics that force is proportional to acceleration, and that if we study the acceleration of some body part, we are getting close to seeing how this remarkable control mechanism produces the movement that we see and feel.

Our capacity for speech is remarkable. In conversation, we can easily pronounce 14 phonemes per second, and this rate appears to be limited by the cognitive aspects of language rather than by the physical ability to perform the articulatory movements. Considering the muscles of the thoracic and abdominal walls, the neck and face, the larynx and pharynx, and the oral cavity, there are over 100 muscles that must be controlled centrally.

Does the brain plan sequences of speech movements as a group, or does it just control each movement in turn without regard to preceding or following phonemes? In speech production, the concept of *coarticulation* implies that the characteristics of each phoneme are adjusted to accommodate aspects of what is coming up ahead.

We can gain some insight into coarticulation by studying the lower lip. The lower lip plays a modest role in speech articulation, but is easily acces-

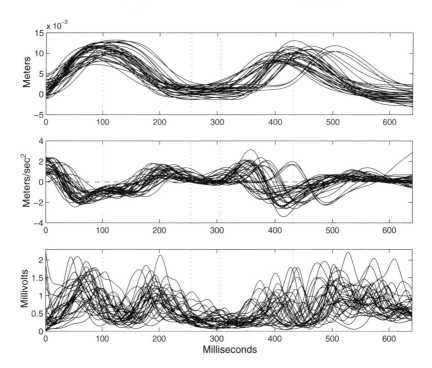

Figure 10.1. The top panel displays the position of the center of the lower lip of a speaker pronouncing the syllable "bob" for 32 replications. The middle panel displays the corresponding accelerations. The bottom panel contains electromyogram (EMG) recordings from a facial muscle that depresses the lower lip, the depressor labii inferior. The dotted lines indicate distinct phases in the articulation of the syllable. The EMG recordings are shifted to the right by 50 milliseconds, the time lag of the direct effect of a neural excitation as a muscle contraction.

sible, and is controlled by only three muscles. We can investigate how these muscles work together to control the lip, and how their contractions are determined by neural activation. We focus on the most important of the three, the depressor labii inferior (DLI) muscle that depresses the lower lip. To produce each /b/, the lip moves up to close the mouth, and then down. During these movements the DLI muscle plays specific roles: one, referred to as *agonist*, when it accelerates the lip during the descending phases, and the other, called *antagonist*, when it brakes the movement during the ascending phases.

Implanting electrodes to observe neural activity directly would involve more heroism than most subjects would consider worthwhile, but we can measure a byproduct of this activity through electromyographical (EMG) recording. Recordings are taken from the surface of the skin, and do not seriously perturb normal movement.

However, there are some issues with EMG recordings as indicators of neural activity. A muscle that is stretched in the absence of neural activation will also generate an EMG signal. Where muscles are overlapping or even just close together, the recording may not cleanly separate activity in different muscles. Finally, there is a period of about 50 msec following the onset of neural excitation, and the associated EMG signal, before muscle contraction begins.

Even if there is some imprecision in whatever EMG reflects, it cannot exert an influence backward in time on lip acceleration, since neural activity shows up in EMG signals with essentially no delay. Consequently we are interested in a *feedforward* model for the influence of EMG on lip acceleration. However, because of the 50 msec lag between neural activation onset and muscle contraction, only associations at delays substantially larger than 50 msec are evidence for coarticulation effects.

10.2   The lip and EMG curves

A subject was repeatedly required to say the syllable "bob," embedded in the phrase, "Say bob again." Because of the delay in muscle contraction indicated above, the records have been shifted in time, dropping the first 50 msec from the observed lip acceleration curves, and the last 50 msec from the raw EMG records. The duration of "bob" in each original record was time-normalized to 690 msec, but because of this time shift, only 640 mscc is displayed in Figure 10.1.

The top panel of Figure 10.1 shows a sample of $N = 32$ trajectories of the lower lip. In the middle panel, the acceleration functions $Y_i(t)$ estimated from these original observations are shown. The bottom panel of Figure 10.1 shows the EMG records. The value $Z_i(s)$ plotted at any particular time s is the recording actually made at time s msec, but the values of lip position and lip acceleration plotted for the same time are those actually observed at time $s + 50$ msec, when any muscle contraction associated with activation at s msec is beginning to take place. Thus, for example, the last EMG observation plotted is for 640 msec, but the actual time for the corresponding lip observations is really 690 msec. For simplicity, we specify lip times from here on as the actual time less 50 msec. However, it is sometimes important to consider the real time of the observations, as we see below.

The lower lip trajectory can be segmented roughly into these epochs, separated by dotted lines in Figure 10.1:

1. close mouth for the first /b/;

2. lower the lip after utterance of first /b/;

3. central part of /o/, lip relatively stationary;

4. raise the lip for second /b/; and

5. lower the lip after the second /b/.

As we noted above, we can expect substantial EMG activity whenever the DLI muscle is active, whether the lip is descending or ascending. The point of least EMG activity is at about 330 milliseconds, at the end of the period when the lip is at its lowest point during the utterance of /o/.

How is the variability across observations of the EMG recording $Z(s)$ reflected in the behavior of the lip acceleration $Y(t)$? It is implausible to suppose that $Z(s)$ acts backward in time to influence $Y(t)$. Examination of Figure 10.1 may suggest that there is some forward influence of EMG activity on lip acceleration, but there is clearly statistical work to be done in investigating this possibility.

As a first step in studying the possible forward influence of EMG activity, we look at the correlation over the 32 replications of the electromyogram at times s and the acceleration at times $t \geq s$. The results are plotted in Figure 10.2. The light and dark patches on or very close to the diagonal of the image indicate a substantial amount of simultaneous relationship of both positive and negative polarity.

We can check for feedforward influence by scanning horizontally, to the left of the diagonal, for a fixed time t. For example, the dashed lines in the figure correspond to about 425 msec, when the lip is closed for the second /b/. We see a patch of positive correlation at about 350 msec; EMG activity 50 msec before this time, during the full opening of the mouth, is correlated with later acceleration. Further back, however, we see some negative correlation at about 175 msec, corresponding to EMG activity during the closure for the first /b/. As we scan parallel to the diagonal, we see a slightly curved band of positive correlation at a lag somewhere around 150 msec, and another band, but of negative correlation, further back at around 200 msec.

10.3   The linear model for the data

Let $T = 640$ indicate the final time of the complete utterance, and let δ be the time lag beyond which we conjecture that there is no influence of EMG activity $Z(s)$ on the lip acceleration $Y(t)$. With this in mind, we model $Z(s)$ as influencing $Y(t)$ according to the model:

$$Y_i(t) = \alpha(t) + \int_{t-\delta}^{t} Z_i(s)\beta(s,t)\,ds + \epsilon_i(t) . \tag{10.1}$$

Here $\alpha(t)$ is a fixed *intercept* function that allows for the relationship between the mean lip and EMG curves, but cannot accommodate their covariation effects. The model presumes that EMG affects lip acceleration

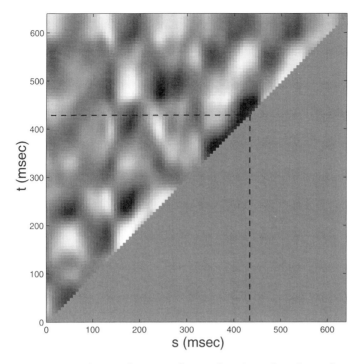

Figure 10.2. The correlations between the accelerations, functions of t, and the electromyogram recordings, functions of s, for all pairs of time values $s \leq t$. White regions correspond to positive correlations and dark regions to negative correlations. The gray level below the diagonal corresponds to a value of zero.

in a linear fashion, and the residual function $\epsilon_i(t)$ reflects the inability of the linear prediction model to fit the data completely. We might call this the *historical linear model* in the sense that the influence of $Z(s)$ feeds forward in time for a time lag of up to δ, and therefore is a relevant part of the history of $Y(t)$ for $s \leq t \leq s + \delta$. Since $s \leq t$, the regression coefficient function $\beta(s, t)$ is defined on a subset of the triangular domain used in Figure 10.2.

By contrast, the pointwise model

$$Y_i(t) = \alpha(t) + Z_i(t)\beta(t) + \epsilon_i(t) , \tag{10.2}$$

could be called *contemporary*, because the influence of EMG on lip acceleration is only instantaneous. In the contemporary model the regression function $\beta(t)$ depends only on t. The model can be viewed as a limiting version of the historical model as $\delta \to 0$.

The central question is, then, whether the contemporary model provides an adequate fit, or whether we should use a model in which β depends on both s and t. If we do fit a historical linear model, then we would also hope to gain some insight into the appropriate value of the lag δ.

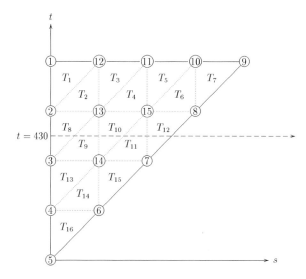

Figure 10.3. The domain of definition of the regression function $\beta(s, t)$ discretized into 16 triangular elements. Element boundaries are indicated by dotted lines and nodes by circled numbers. As an illustration, the horizontal dashed line at $t = 430$ represents the line of integration for $Y_r(430)$.

10.4   The estimated regression function

A practical approach to the estimation of the regression function $\beta(s, t)$ is to seek an expansion in terms of a fixed number of known basis functions. We use the *finite element method*, often used in engineering to solve partial differential equation systems. This approach involves subdividing the domain $(s, t), s \leq t$, into triangular regions in the manner shown in Figure 10.3. The triangles are called the *elements* and the vertices of the triangles are called the *nodes* of the system. Sixteen triangles are shown in the figure, corresponding to four intervals along each axis; but our final triangulation involved 169 elements and 105 nodes, resulting from using 13 intervals along each axis, each interval being of length $640/13 = 49.2$ msec.

The next step is to define basis functions over each of these regions. Each basis function $\phi_k(s, t)$ is a linear bivariate function having the value one at a specific node and falling off to zero at the remote edges of each triangle that has that node as a vertex. A typical basis function for a node inside the triangular domain is shown in Figure 10.4.

The triangular basis has an important advantage in considering how large the lag δ should be in modeling the feedforward influence of $Z(s)$. Triangles falling more than δ units from the diagonal are simply eliminated, so that the manipulation of δ corresponds to selecting subsets of the basis functions. Of course, we can only set δ at discrete values, but this is not a problem if we make the triangular mesh reasonably fine. Letting Δ indicate the width

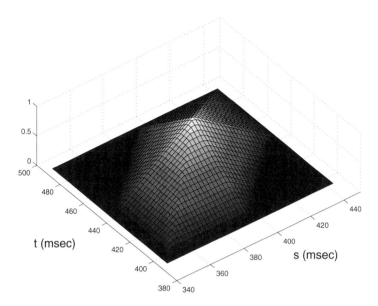

Figure 10.4. A typical piecewise linear basis function used to construct a finite element approximation of the regression function $\beta(s,t)$.

of a single triangle, we are permitted to use lag values $\delta = m\Delta$ for integers $m \geq 1$.

The contemporary model (10.2) can be thought of as the case $m = 0$. In this case, the elements are intervals along the diagonal line. The basis functions are functions of only one variable t, and are piecewise linear functions, in other words, B-splines of order 2, as shown in Figure 2.14.

Once we have estimated the coefficients b_k, we have a piecewise linear approximation to the regression function $\beta(s,t)$. The process of estimating the coefficients of the expansion can be set up as a matrix computation; for further details, see Malfait, Ramsay, and Froda (2001).

Figure 10.5 shows the full bivariate regression function $\beta(s,t)$, effectively setting $\delta = T$, as a grayscale image. For what values of t is lip acceleration most influenced by current and previous EMG activity? We see that the patterns of relationship that we already observed in Figure 10.2 are also found here, but the regression function surface is much better at picking out specific intervals where the influence is important. The peaks and dips in $\beta(s,t)$ indicate that the lip activity is most influenced by measured EMG in the time interval from about $t = 350$ to about $t = 480$, the time of the second lip closure. By scanning along the line corresponding to 425 msec, we note that there is also some indication that EMG activity at time $t = 250$, at the beginning of /o/, influences the second /b/ closure.

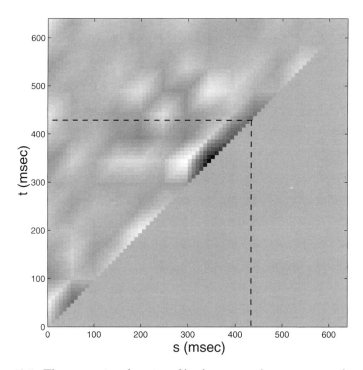

Figure 10.5. The regression function $\beta(s,t)$ estimated using 105 nodes. Dark regions correspond to negative values and white regions to positive values. The gray level plotted below the diagonal corresponds to the value zero.

10.5   How far back should the historical model go?

What lag δ seems to be supported by the data? To answer this, we need to compare a fit for a specific lag to that offered by a simpler, and more restricted, model. Two simpler models are the mean computed across the 32 replications,

$$\bar{Y}(t) = N^{-1} \sum_{i=1}^{32} Y_i(t) \,,$$

and the contemporary model (10.2).

For a specific $\delta = m\Delta$, we can define the error sum of squares function at any time t by

$$\text{SSE}_m(t) = \sum_{i=1}^{N} \{Y_i(t) - \hat{Y}_i(t)\}^2, \qquad (10.3)$$

where $\hat{Y}_i(t)$ is the fit of the current model to the observed curve $Y_i(t)$. For any given value of m, the squared multiple correlation measure of fit R_m^2

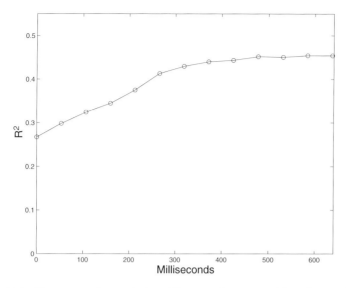

Figure 10.6. The squared correlation R_m^2 as a function of lag $\delta = m\Delta$ for a triangulation into 169 elements and 105 nodes. The points plotted correspond to the discrete values of δ given by integers m.

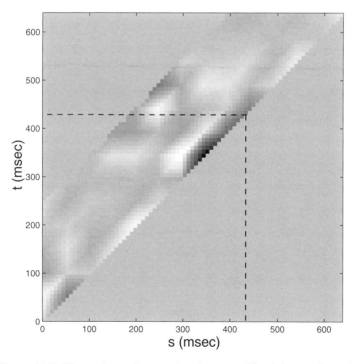

Figure 10.7. The estimated regression function $\beta(s, t)$ for lag $\delta = 5\Delta$.

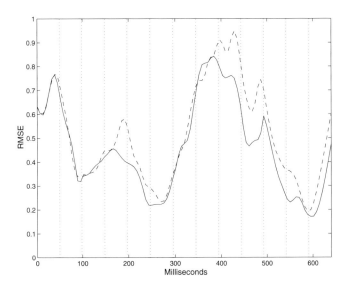

Figure 10.8. The error function RMSE(t) for the models with lag $\delta = 5\Delta \approx 250$ (solid line) and $\delta = 0$ (dashed line). The vertical dotted lines indicate the positions on the axis of the nodes of the finite element basis.

is defined by

$$R_m^2 = 1 - \frac{\int_0^T \mathrm{SSE}_m(t)\, dt}{\int_0^T \mathrm{SSY}(t)\, dt}, \qquad (10.4)$$

where SSY(t) refers to the fit using the mean curve.

We consider R_m^2 as a function of $\delta = m\Delta$, that is, as a function of the width of the domain of integration in the model (10.1). From Figure 10.6, we see that the fit improves as we enlarge the domain of integration up to $\delta = 5\Delta$, but does not increase substantially with larger values of δ. Thus, it seems to be worth modeling lip acceleration at time t to be influenced by EMG values up to about 250 msec before t. The estimate of $\beta(s, t)$ using this lag is shown in Figure 10.7.

The shape of the estimate of $\beta(s, t)$ indicates, as expected from the regression function already considered, that the muscle activation is the most influential in the period leading up to the second lip closure times. Also, there is a ridge of influence along the diagonal continuing for a short period after the closure; in this short interval it is only contemporary EMG signals that matter. This suggests that the system plans the closure, but the recovery after the closure is not planned for in advance.

Figure 10.8 compares the standard deviation function RMSE(t) = $\sqrt{\mathrm{SSE}_m(t)/N}$ for the historical model with $m = 5$ with that for the contemporary model $m = 0$. We see that the main improvement for the historical model is in the articulation of the second /b/ between 400 and 500 msec, and also more briefly at about 200 msec, in the transition from the first /b/ to the /o/ phoneme.

Is the fit of the historical model with $m = 5$ significantly better than that of the contemporary model? Because different finite element bases are used to approximate the two models, the finite element contemporary model is not exactly nested within the finite element historical model, even though the exact models can be regarded as nested. In order to compare nested models, therefore, we approximate the contemporary model by the historical model with $m = 1$, and construct an F-test of significance. Results reported in full in Malfait, Ramsay, and Froda (2001) then demonstrate that the fit of the model with $m = 5$ is indeed significantly better than the approximate contemporary model $m = 1$.

10.6   What have we seen?

It now seems fairly clear from these results that the timing and intensity of phonemes do have a covariation with EMG activity that is reflected both in the simple correlation plot in Figure 10.2, and in the feedforward linear model (10.1). The time lag over which this feedforward influence is evident is not unlimited, and in this case corresponds to two phonemes. Of this 250 msec lag, we are able to account for 45% of the variation in $Y(t)$ by its covariation with $Z(s)$. This is a substantial effect, considering how volatile EMG data tend to be, as well as their tentative connection with neural activity. The pointwise or contemporary linear model only explains about 27% of the variability, and Figure 10.8 indicates that its deficiency as a model seems mainly concentrated on the second "b," where the feedforward influence is especially strong.

Ramsay and Silverman (1997, Chapters 9 to 11) give a general introduction to functional linear models, and discuss various aspects in more detail. However, their treatment does not go as far as the restriction of the influence to a finite lag, and the present case study exemplifies the way that functional data analysis methods often have to be tailored to the particular problem under consideration. The finite element method adopted was particularly appropriate to the restriction to finite lag on the triangular domain over which $\beta(s, t)$ is defined. This approach also allowed a simple control of the size of the lag δ so that we could explore the role of this parameter.

10.7   Notes and bibliography

The data were collected at the Haskins Speech Laboratories at Yale University by V. Gracco. The analyses of the data were carried out by N.

Nicole during a Masters of Science program at the Université du Québec at Montréal, and reported in more detail in Malfait, Ramsay, and Froda (2001).

The raw lip position data consisted of two-dimensional positions in the sagittal plane sampled 625 times per second. Jaw position was also recorded, and subtracted from lip position. Although two-dimensional position measurements were taken, in fact the trajectory of the lower lip was nearly linear, and consequently the data were reduced to one-dimensional coordinates by principal components analysis.

A considerable amount of preliminary processing was required before satisfactory acceleration curves could be produced. The data were first smoothed by a robust method, the LOWESS smoother (Cleveland, 1979) in the S-PLUS package to eliminate the occasional outlying recording. These smoothed data were in turn approximated using 100 B-spline basis functions. The spline basis was of order 6 in order to assure that the second derivative of the expansion would be reasonably smooth. A light roughness penalty on the fourth derivative was applied in order to smooth the second derivative further.

The EMG data were sampled at 1250 hertz, and were much noisier than position records, showing very high frequency oscillations about zero as well as the slower trends that interest us. As is usual for EMG measures, the raw data were replaced by values of a linear envelope of the absolute values. These values were then further smoothed.

The contemporary model (10.2) can be viewed as a functional extension of the *varying coefficient model* of Hastie and Tibshirani (1993).

11

The Dynamics of Handwriting Printed Characters

11.1 Recording handwriting in real time

The way we handwrite characters is a deeply individual matter, as bank tellers who ask for your signature and graphologists who claim to be able to study your personality from your handwriting know well. The handwriting samples that they work with are static, in the sense that they consider the trace left behind well after the signature is formed, and thus are at one remove from the person who actually did the original writing. In this sense, any attempts to identify an individual, let alone to claim to reconstruct aspects of their personalities, have the flavor of archaeological digs.

What if we could use the online time course of the formation of a signature? Would we not see things as the signature unfolds in time that could not be observed in the static image? Could we see, for example, when a person was nervous, in a hurry, suffering from the onset of Parkinsonism, or rejoicing in a state of profound tranquillity and peace? Surely we could discover new ways by which a handwriting sample characterizes a specific individual, and perhaps use this to make forgery harder than it is now.

In this chapter we use what we call a dynamic model for handwriting. We demonstrate how the model can be fitted to the writing of a particular individual using repeated samples of their printing. We also investigate how well the model separates one person from another.

Our first task, however, is a brief and nontechnical account of some simple dynamic models. Those familiar with differential equations may well be happy to skip ahead, but many readers will find this next section important.

11.2   An introduction to dynamic models

The term *dynamic* implies change. When we speak of the dynamics of a function of time, we are discussing some aspect of the change in curve values over small changes in time, and we therefore focus on one or more of the derivatives of the curve. Chapter 6 described the dynamics of growth, and indeed we defined growth there as the rate of change of height.

A dynamic model therefore involves one or more derivatives with respect to time. Because a number of orders of derivatives may be involved, we use the notation $D^m x(t)$ to denote the mth derivative of the function $x(t)$. This is more convenient than using a separate symbol for each derivative, as we did in Chapter 6, or the classic notation

$$\frac{d^m x}{dt^m},$$

which is too typographically bulky to perpetuate here.

The most common form of dynamic model is an equation linking two or more orders of derivatives. In our present notation, the fundamental equation of growth that we developed in Chapter 6 is

$$D^2 x(t) = \beta(t) D x(t), \tag{11.1}$$

and this equation links the first derivative to the second by the functional factor $\beta(t)$. It is an example of a *linear* differential equation and has the structure of a standard regression model, albeit one expressed in functional terms:

- the acceleration $D^2 x(t)$ is the dependent variable,

- the velocity $D x(t)$ is the independent variable,

- $\beta(t)$ is the regression coefficient, and

- the residual or error, not shown in the model (11.1), is zero.

The regression model is functional in that the variables and the coefficient $\beta(t)$ all depend on t. But if we fix time t, and we have in hand N replications $x_i(t)$ of the curve, you can well imagine that ordinary regression analysis would be one practical way to estimate the value of $\beta(t)$ at a fixed time t_j. As the dependent variable in a standard regression, you would use the N values $y_i = D^2 x_i(t_j)$ for $i = 1, \ldots, N$. The corresponding independent variable values would be $z_i = D x_i(t_j)$, and so you would estimate the constant $\beta(t_j)$ as the coefficient $b = \sum y_i z_i / \sum z_i^2$ resulting from regressing y on z without an intercept. And you would be quite right!

We briefly review how a differential equation determines the behavior of a function, by considering a second-order linear differential equation, restricted to having constant coefficients:

$$D^2 x(t) = \beta_0 x(t) + \beta_1 D x(t). \tag{11.2}$$

Table 11.1. Some processes defined by a second-order linear differential equation with constant coefficients

Process	Equation	Coefficients	
		β_0	β_1
Linear motion	$x(t) = a + bt$	0	0
Exponential growth/decay	$x(t) = a + be^{\gamma t}$	0	γ
Harmonic motion	$x(t) = a\sin\omega t + b\cos\omega t$	$-\omega^2$	0
Damped harmonic motion	$x(t) = e^{\gamma t}(a\sin\omega t + b\cos\omega t)$	$-\omega^2$	γ

Table 11.1 relates some special cases of the equation to some familiar functional models and physical processes.

The constants a and b in the table are arbitrary. We see that equation (11.2) covers three basic dynamic processes of science. If both coefficients are zero, we have the linear motion exhibited by bodies that are free of any external force. But if $-\beta_0$ is a positive number, we see the other type of stationary motion, that of perpetual oscillation.[1] Introducing a nonzero value for β_1, however, results in exponential growth or decay, without oscillation if $\beta_0 = 0$, and superimposed on harmonic motion otherwise.

Note, too, the models in Table 11.1 also define the simultaneous behavior of a certain number of derivatives. In fact, the characteristics of both the first and second derivatives are essentially specialized versions of the behaviors of the functions themselves. In this sense, then, these models are really about the dynamics of the processes.

In (11.2) we considered the special case of constant coefficients. What difference does it make if the coefficients $\beta_0(t)$ and $\beta_1(t)$ also change with time? If the change is not rapid, we can consider the corresponding differential equation as describing a system that has an evolving dynamics, in the sense that its frequency of oscillation and its rate of exponential growth or decay are themselves changing through time. The larger the value of $-\beta_0(t)$ the more rapidly the system will oscillate near time t.

In this chapter and subsequently, we use linear differential equation models of order m in the general form

$$D^m x(t) = \alpha(t) + \sum_{j=0}^{m-1} \beta_j(t)D^j x(t). \tag{11.3}$$

There are m coefficient functions $\beta_j(t)$ that define the equations, but in specific applications we may want to fix the values of some of these. In particular we may set one or more to zero.

---

[1] Coefficient $-\beta_0$ can also be negative, of course, and in this case the sines and cosines in the last two rows of Table 11.1 must be replaced by their hyperbolic counterparts. But the positive case is seen much more often in applications.

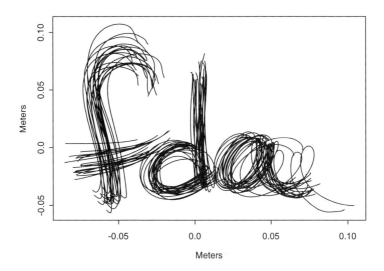

Figure 11.1. Twenty registered printings of the characters "fda."

In addition to the coefficients $\beta_j(t)$, the form (11.3) contains the function $\alpha(t)$, called the *forcing function* in many fields that use differential equations. The function $\alpha(t)$ often reflects external or exogenous influences on the system not captured by the main part of the equation, or that part of the derivative $D^m x(t)$ not captured by the simultaneous variation in the lower-order derivatives. From a regression analysis perspective, we may regard $\alpha(t)$ as the constant or intercept term. If $\alpha(t) = 0$, the differential equation is said to be *homogeneous*, and otherwise is *nonhomogeneous*.

11.3   One subject's printing data

The data are the X-, Y- and Z-coordinates of the tip of the pen captured 200 times a second while one subject, designated "JR," prints the characters "fda" $N = 20$ times. The X-coordinate is the left-to-right position on the writing surface. Coordinate Y is the up-and-down position on the writing surface, and Z is the position upward from the writing surface. Of course, static records give very little information about Z at all—we can only see the X and Y values corresponding to times when Z is zero, and at times when Z is nonzero we have no data at all. The additional richness of a dynamic record is considerable.

Extensive preprocessing is required before we are ready to fit a differential equation. The times of the beginning of "f" and the end of "a" for each

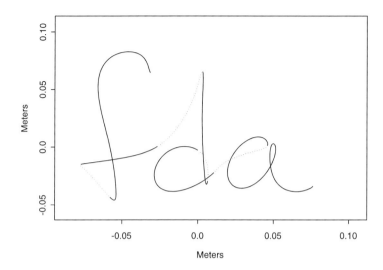

Figure 11.2. The average of 20 registered printings of "fda." The average position of the pen was on or very near the writing surface for the solid lines, and lifted off for the dotted lines.

record must be identified, and the coordinate system in which measurements were taken must be rotated and translated to the (X, Y, Z) system that we described above. In addition we register, or time-warp, the records $[x_i(t), y_i(t), z_i(t)], i = 1, \ldots, N$ to a common template $[x_0(t), y_0(t), z_0(t)]$. The details of the registration step are described in Chapter 7, and we assume that we can take off from where we left the handwriting problem there. Figure 11.1 shows the trace in the X–Y plane of the 20 functional records, after registration.

Figure 11.2 displays the mean characters for this subject. Most of the registration process does not affect the individual static records plotted in Figure 11.1, but, as we saw in Chapter 6, registration is crucial in the estimation of the mean. The regions where the average position of the pen is clearly above the writing surface are shown in Figure 11.2 as dotted lines, and we see that there are four such intervals. The characters are formed from five strokes on the writing surface (two for "f," two for "d," and one for "a") along with the four off the surface. The average time taken to print these characters was 2.345 seconds, and corresponds to an average of 0.26 seconds per stroke. Note the two sudden changes of direction or cusps between the main part of the "f" and its cross-stroke, and at the beginning and end of the downstroke for "d." There is a lot of energy in such sudden events, and they may be hard for a dynamic model to capture.

11.4   A differential equation for handwriting

We now want to estimate a linear differential equation for each of the three coordinate functions. We use a third-order equation, $m = 3$. The third derivative is sometimes called "jerk."

To make our task a bit easier, we simplify our equation by fixing $\beta_0(t) = 0$. Without this constraint, the equation would have to be recalibrated for any translation of the coordinate values. The resulting equation is, in the case of the X-coordinate for record i,

$$D^3 x_i(t) = \alpha_x(t) + \beta_{x1}(t) D x_i(t) + \beta_{x2}(t) D^2 x_i(t) + \epsilon_{xi}(t). \qquad (11.4)$$

There are two coefficient functions $\beta_{x1}(t)$ and $\beta_{x2}(t)$, as well as the forcing or intercept function $\alpha_x(t)$. In effect, this is a second-order nonhomogeneous linear differential equation in pen velocity, so we can think of velocity as our basic observed variable. The residual function $\epsilon_{xi}(t)$ varies from replicate to replicate, and represents variation in the third derivative in each curve that is not accounted for by the model. There are, of course, corresponding coefficient, forcing, and residual functions associated with coordinates Y and Z. In particular, the forcing function for coordinate Z is the aspect that allows the pen to lift off the paper, because when the pen is in contact with the paper z_i and all its derivatives are zero.

We carry out one additional preprocessing step, by removing the linear trend in the X-coordinate as the hand moves from left to right. In effect, this positions the origin for X in a moving coordinate frame that can be thought of as at the center of the wrist. If the slope of the linear trend is v, the adjusted X-coordinate will satisfy the same model as the original, with a multiple of $v\beta_{x1}$ added to the forcing function. So this linear correction will only have an important effect on the model if there is substantial variability in the rate of moving from left to right, which in practice there is not.

How do we estimate an equation such as (11.4)? Our first task is to find a good nonparametric estimate of the derivative functions using the 20 replications. These function estimates are then used to estimate the two coefficient functions $\beta_{x1}(t)$ and $\beta_{x2}(t)$ and the forcing function $\alpha_x(t)$. Returning to the regression perspective, a successful equation will mean that the residual function $\epsilon_{xi}(t)$ is relatively small for all records and all t. The natural approach will be ordinary least squares in the sense that we choose to minimize, in the X-coordinate case,

$$\text{SSE}_X = \sum_{i=1}^{N} \int_0^T \epsilon_{xi}^2(t)\, dt.$$

The adequacy of the fit can be assessed by comparing the residuals to the third derivative, which acts as the dependent variable in the regression analysis. The technique for minimizing SSE_X with respect to $\alpha_x(t)$, $\beta_{x1}(t)$, and

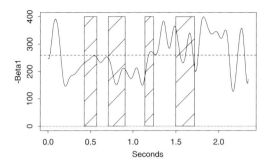

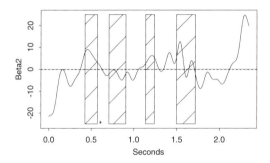

Figure 11.3. The top panel shows the function $-\beta_{x1}(t)$ for the differential equation describing the motion of the pen in the horizontal or X direction. The dashed-dotted line indicates the average value, and corresponds to a horizontal oscillation every 0.58 seconds. The bottom panel shows the corresponding function $\beta_{x2}(t)$, and this tends to oscillate about zero. It controls the instantaneous exponential growth or decay in the instantaneous oscillation. The shaded areas correspond to periods when the pen is lifted off the paper.

$\beta_{x2}(t)$ was developed by Ramsay (1996b), who called the method *principal differential analysis* because of its close conceptual relationship to principal component analysis.

Figure 11.3 displays the two estimated coefficient functions for the X-coordinate. Although it is hard to see much to interpret in these functions, one can compare them to the equation for harmonic motion in Table 11.1. We notice immediately that there is considerable variability in both functions about the average value, also displayed in the plot. This variability is due to the control of the hand by the contracting and relaxing muscles, and these in turn are controlled by neural activation arriving from the motor cortex of the brain. The rapid local variations in the plots are easily ignored "by eye," but perhaps suggest that a regularization term could be

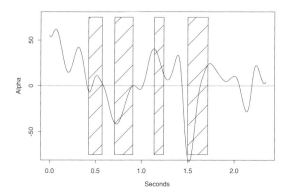

Figure 11.4. The forcing function $\alpha_x(t)$ for the differential equation describing the motion of the pen in the horizontal or X direction. The dashed-dotted line indicates the average value of the third derivative, to give an idea of the relative size of $\alpha_x(t)$. Episodes of forcing occur when $\alpha_x(t)$ deviates strongly from zero. The shaded areas correspond to periods when the pen is lifted off the paper.

added to the criterion SSE_X. The formal inclusion of regularization is an interesting topic for future investigation.

Function $-\beta_{x1}(t)$ plays the role of ω^2 in the harmonic equation and, since the period of oscillation in a harmonic system is $2\pi/\omega$, the larger the value of $\beta_{x1}(t)$ at some time point t, the faster the velocity is oscillating at that time. The average value of $-\beta_{x1}(t)$ is 259, corresponding to an oscillation every $2\pi/\sqrt{259} = 0.39$ seconds. This means that the hand is producing a horizontal stroke once each 0.20 seconds, on the average, which agrees closely with what we observed in Figure 11.2.

On the other hand, coefficient function $\beta_2(t)$ varies about a value relatively close to zero. It determines the instantaneous exponential growth $(\beta_{x2}(t) > 0)$ or decay $(\beta_{x2}(t) < 0)$ in the oscillations.

Corresponding analyses were performed for the other two coordinates. The dynamics of the Y-coordinate resemble those of the X-coordinate, in that the average value of $-\beta_{y2}(t)$ is 277, and this also corresponds to a period of about 0.38 seconds. The Z-coordinate, however, has an average period of 0.29 seconds.

Figure 11.4 shows the estimated forcing function $\alpha_x(t)$ for the X-coordinate. We focus our attention on times when $\alpha_x(t)$ deviates strongly from zero, indicating times when the homogeneous version of the equation will not capture the intensity of the dynamics. The first peak is in the curved part of the "f" downstroke, when the pen is changing direction and probably accelerating. The next substantial deviation coincides with the pen leaving the paper to cross over to begin the "d" downstroke. There is

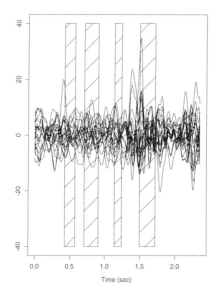

Figure 11.5. The residual functions $\epsilon_{xi}(t)$ for the X-coordinate. Shaded areas indicate periods when the pen is off the writing surface.

another forced point at the cusp at the end of the "d" downstroke, again just as the pen leaves the writing surface to begin the loop part of "d." We see the largest deviation as the pen leaves the writing surface to cross over to begin "a." In summary, forcing events coincide either with points of sharp curvature or cusps, or with the pen leaving the writing surface. The change in the frictional forces as the pen leaves the surface seems to be an important part of the dynamics.

11.5   Assessing the fit of the equation

Now we want to see how well this equation fits the data. One way to do this is to work with the regression concept, and calculate the squared multiple correlation measure, or proportion of variability explained,

$$R_X^2 = 1 - \frac{\sum_{i=1}^{N} \int_0^T \epsilon_{xi}^2(t)\, dt}{\sum_{i=1}^{N} \int_0^T D^3 x_i^2(t)\, dt}. \tag{11.5}$$

The values we obtain are 0.991, 0.994, and 0.994 for the X-, Y-, and Z-coordinates, respectively, indicating a very good fit in all three cases.

As the value of R_X^2 indicates, the residual functions are much smaller overall than the original third derivatives $D^3 x_i$. However, integrating across time in (11.5) risks missing something interesting that might occur at some specific points in time. Figure 11.5 plots the 20 residual functions for the X-coordinate, and we see that these are small relative to the size of the third derivative, and that they are concentrated around zero. They seem to behave as random "noise" functions that do not contain any systematic variability that we have failed to fit. This investigation shows that the dynamic model generally fits the data extremely well, and invites the suggestion that the coefficient functions characterize the particular subject in some way, and hence can be used as the basis of a classification method in preference to direct consideration of the handwriting itself. This is the theme of our next section.

However, we do notice that there are some sharp excursions in the forcing functions, with a couple of the largest being associated with the beginnings of intervals when the pen is off the paper. It may be that the change in frictional forces plus the effect of raising the pen can have a noticeable effect on printing dynamics in the X–Y plane. Maybe things would be simpler if we only used cursive handwriting, and you can consult Ramsay (2000) to compare these results with that situation.

11.6   Classifying writers by using their dynamic equations

We can now estimate a linear differential equation to describe the data of different people printing the same characters. How well does one person's equation model another person's data? We now introduce a second subject, called "CC," and consider a set of 20 replications of CC's printing of the characters "fda." In order to ensure that both dynamic models are defined on compatible time scales, CC's data are preprocessed by being registered to the mean curve of the registered JR data. Thus all the data are registered to the same template. After this preprocessing step, a dynamic model for CC's printing is estimated in the way set out above. We now apply the equation for subjects JR and CC to the data for themselves[2] and for each other.

Figure 11.6 shows the X-coordinate residual functions $\epsilon_{xi}(t)$ resulting from applying the equation for subjects JR and CC to both sets of data. Corresponding results for the Y-coordinate are shown in Figure 11.7. What we see in the figures is that the residual functions are much larger, and

---

[2]In the case where the equation is applied to the subject's own data, we reestimated the equation 20 times by dropping each record out in turn, estimating the equation for the remainder of the data, and then applying the equation to the excluded record. This standard leaving-one-out procedure gives a more honest estimate of how the equation will work in practice than the approach where the test record is included in the estimating set.

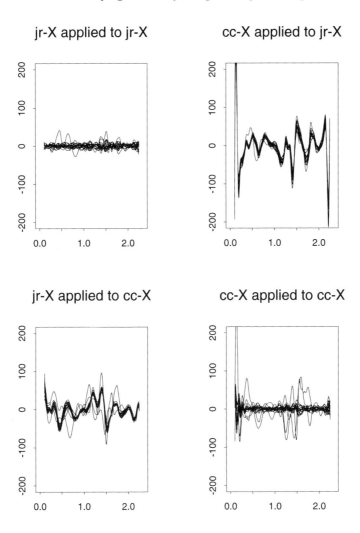

Figure 11.6. The residual functions for the X-coordinate resulting from applying both JR's and CC's differential operators to both sets of data.

also have strong systematic patterns, when they result from applying the equation estimated for one person to the data of the other. The self-applied residual functions for JR are rather smaller than those for CC, and two of the CC curves yield self-applied residual functions that are considerably larger in places. Subject CC seems to have altered his printing style in some important respect in these two anomalous cases. Thus, this technology also may be useful for detecting when people alter in some fundamental way how they print or write a sequence of characters.

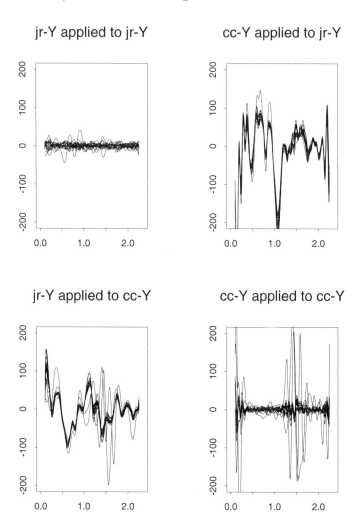

Figure 11.7. The residual functions for the Y-coordinate resulting from applying both JR's and CC's differential operators to both sets of data.

Figure 11.8 investigates a simple numerical summary based on these results. We assessed the magnitude of the residual functions by computing the square root of their average squared values. As well as averaging across time, we average across all three coordinates in order to obtain a single number quantifying the residuals in Figures 11.6 and 11.7 and the corresponding residuals for the Z-coordinate. The figure uses box plots to show the distribution of these magnitudes for the four situations. We see that the JR operators decisively separate the magnitudes for the two subjects'

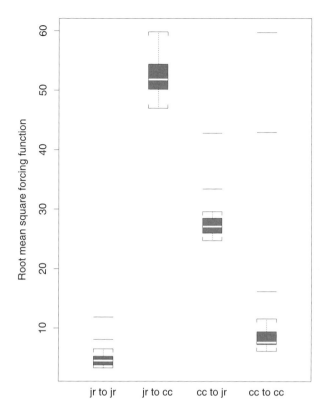

Figure 11.8. Box plots of the root mean square magnitudes of the residual functions resulting from applying both JR's and CC's differential operators to both sets of data. For each replication, the root mean square is calculated taking the average over time and all three coordinates.

printing. The largest value for JR's own data is about 12, and the smallest value for CC's data is about 45.

When the CC operators are used, the subtlety of the data becomes clearer. Using a cutoff value of 20, say, the 18 nonanomalous CC printings are clearly separated from the JR printings. On the other hand, the two anomalous printings are very badly modeled by the CC operators (estimated each time leaving out the individual datum in question). If we were using this simple numerical summary to classify the data, we would presumably categorize these two data as being written by neither CC or JR. If we look back to Figure 11.7, however, we can see that even the two anomalous curves yield residual curves that are near zero over the part of the range $[0.3, 1.2]$. We do not pursue this further in the present study, but it demonstrates that attempts to fool the dynamic model may not always be totally successful on closer examination.

11.7   What have we seen?

The methods of functional data analysis are especially well suited to studying the dynamics of processes that interest us. We saw this previously in our phase-plane plotting of the nondurable goods index, and now we see that a differential equation is a useful means of modeling this time-varying behavior. Of course, this is already well known in the natural sciences, where differential equations, such as Maxwell's equations for electromagnetic phenomena, emerge as the most elegant and natural means of expressing the laws of physics and chemistry.

But in the natural sciences differential equations emerged painstakingly after much experimentation and observation, and finally some deep thinking about the way the interplay of forces along with the law of conservation of energy might determine the results of these experiments. Now, however, we are evolving methods for estimating these equations directly from often noisy data, and in situations such as economics and biomechanics where fundamental laws will not be straightforward and may not even be possible. In this chapter we have put our empirically estimated differential equations to work to investigate an interesting practical problem, the identification of an individual by the dynamic characteristics of a sample of his or her behavior. The next chapter applies this idea to some rather more complex biomechanical data.

12
A Differential Equation for Juggling

12.1   Introduction

Chapter 11 introduced the notion of modeling functional data using a differential equation. We introduced this type of model by relating it to ordinary least squares regression analysis. In this chapter we tackle a similar problem, but in a more challenging context that requires some extensions of the approach.

We saw that a sample of handwriting could be described by a linear differential equation of the form

$$x'''(t) = \beta_1(t)x'(t) + \beta_2(t)x''(t) + f(t) , \qquad (12.1)$$

where $x'(t)$ is velocity, $x''(t)$ is acceleration, $x'''(t)$ is the third derivative or jerk taken along a specific coordinate direction, and $f(t)$ is a forcing or residual term that we hope is small. In the handwriting data, we had a separate equation of this sort for each of three coordinates, with the X-axis along the line of writing, the Y-axis vertically on the paper, and the Z-coordinate measuring a lift off the paper.

What makes a differential equation model particularly interesting is its capacity to link the observed position function $x(t)$ in a particular coordinate direction with the behavior of the velocity, acceleration and jerk functions, which we must derive from the observed data. It is at the level of acceleration especially that we can expect to see the influence of the body's motor control system, as contracting muscles apply forces to the body's framework, which in turn change acceleration directly as a consequence of Newton's Second Law. However, while the visual system can feed position information back to the brain to modify the control process, in rapid and highly automated tasks such as handwriting and juggling, the time delays involved in neural transmission and central processing imply that visual feedback is playing only a limited role. Instead, the brain probably uses information from the strains applied to the body as it moves and interacts with its environment, and these messages are translated into control over acceleration through muscle contractions. In short, it is at the acceleration level that most of the action is to be found, and a model that accurately couples acceleration with the observable data is vital.

The X-, Y-, and Z-axes defined above constitute the coordinate system used to describe handwriting. Is this coordinate system natural? It is obvious that the X–Y plane should be the plane of the paper, and writing has a preferred direction on the paper, so defining the X-axis to be parallel to the lines on the paper is a natural coordinate system for handwriting. The presence of a natural coordinate system and the lack of external forces (other than the constraint that writing has to be on the paper itself!) must surely simplify the modeling process.

The process of juggling a ball seems more challenging than handwriting, and certainly far fewer people master it. The motion of the hand is in all three dimensions in space, however these dimensions are defined. Moreover, once the ball leaves the hand, the laws of physics take over, and the brain must anticipate where these laws are going to deliver the ball back into the juggler's hand. Since no two throws can be exactly the same, there is inevitably an interaction between brain processes and the external world that may complicate the situation. Finally, it is much less obvious how we should arrange the coordinate axes—or even whether we should use rigid Euclidean coordinates at all. This means that the model must be sufficiently invariant with respect to choice of coordinate frame that the fit will still work even when the statistical analysis has used the "wrong" coordinates.

12.2   The data and preliminary analyses

The data were collected from Professor Michael Newton of the Department of Biostatistics at the University of Wisconsin who, in addition to being a fine statistician, is an expert juggler. He juggled three balls for 10 sequences of 10 seconds each. Within a sequence, there were 12 to 13 cycles of throwing a ball and catching another, with a total of 123 cycles.

Small infrared emitting diodes (IREDs) were placed on the tip of Michael's forefinger, his wrist, and three locations on his chest. The positions of these IREDs were tracked 200 times a second by an OPTOTRAK camera system. Our main concentration is on the data for the tip of the forefinger. The chest IREDs provided a point of reference for slow movements of his entire body, and by subtracting their positions from the other two, these drifts were removed from the data. We used a coordinate system with the X-axis sideways to Michael's right, the Y-axis outward from his body, and the Z-axis vertically upward. In most of our discussion we refer to the X-, Y-, and Z-coordinates as coordinates 1, 2, and 3 respectively.

The data were centered so that the average position was zero for each coordinate. Because we knew that we would need a smooth estimate of the third derivative, the jerk function $x'''(t)$, the data were smoothed using a roughness penalty method penalizing for the integral of the squared fifth derivative of each coordinate function. Software details, together with the data themselves, are given on the Web site corresponding to this chapter. The OPTOTRAK measurements are accurate to within 0.5 mm, and it was appropriate to choose a rather small penalty parameter value of $\lambda = 10^{-12}$.

Here is our notation. The function $x_j(t), j = 1, 2, 3$ indicates the position of the forefinger in the $X, Y,$ and Z directions, respectively. Corresponding velocities are denoted by $x'_j(t)$, accelerations by $x''_j(t)$, and jerks by $x'''_j(t)$. We also need the tangential velocity and the tangential acceleration

$$\|x'(t)\| = \sqrt{x'_1(t)^2 + x'_2(t)^2 + x'_3(t)^2}$$

$$\|x''(t)\| = \sqrt{x''_1(t)^2 + x''_2(t)^2 + x''_3(t)^2} \,. \tag{12.2}$$

Partial cycles at the beginning and end of each record were trimmed off to obtain records that were comparable across trials, and we had to find a suitable landmark or curve feature to separate one cycle from another. The tangential velocity for the finger IRED showed a deep and stable minimum within each cycle, corresponding to the lowest point in the forefinger's trajectory, and the beginning of the launch of the ball. The beginning of a cycle was therefore defined by the location of this minimal value of $\|x'(t)\|$. The average duration of the cycles was 719 msec, and half the durations fell in the interval from 696 to 736 msec. The cycles did show some phase variation, so we applied the continuous registration method described in Section 7.6.1 to the tangential velocity functions $\|x'(t)\|$. The registration process means that averages of the curves and their derivatives will give good summaries of what is happening.

12.3 Features in the average cycle

Figure 12.1 shows the average position of the index finger in terms of coordinates 1 and 3, as could be observed by someone seeing through the juggler from behind. Figure 12.2 displays the view of the cycle from the right of the juggler. It is clear that there is a substantial twist in the cycle, and so all three coordinates are essential.

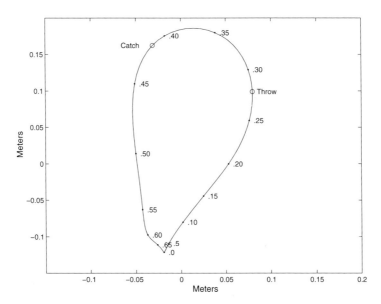

Figure 12.1. The average juggling cycle in the X–Z plane, or as seen from the juggler's perspective facing forward. The points on the curve indicate times in seconds, and the total cycle takes 0.711 seconds. The time when the ball leaves the hand and the time of the catch are shown as circles.

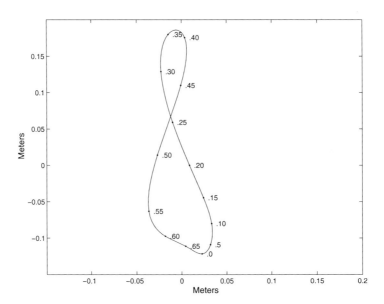

Figure 12.2. The average juggling cycle in the Y–Z plane, as seen from the perspective of someone standing to the juggler's right.

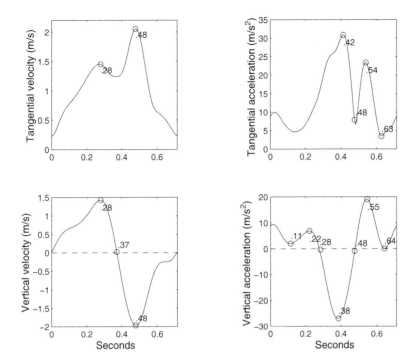

Figure 12.3. The tangential velocity $\|x'(t)\|$ of the tip of the forefinger is shown in the top left panel, and the tangential acceleration $\|x''(t)\|$ is shown in the top right panel. The vertical velocity $x_3'(t)$ and acceleration $x_3''(t)$ of the tip of the forefinger are shown in the bottom left and right panels, respectively. Important features in these curves are indicated by circles, and their times are indicated in seconds.

The cycle begins at the bottom of the trajectory, where the forefinger is poised to begin the launch of the ball. The ball leaves the hand at the point where the motion is nearly vertical, at 0.28 seconds. The catch occurs at 0.42 seconds, after the hand has moved through the top of the arc, and a little before the motion becomes vertical. The ball is lowered to a position a little to the left of the beginning of the cycle, and then transferred laterally to the point where the cycle begins again.

The top two panels in Figure 12.3 display the average tangential velocity and acceleration. We need to also look at the vertical component of acceleration separately since it is the upward movement of the ball that is the key to a successful juggling cycle, and these are found in the bottom two panels. The throw accelerates the ball from near rest to a velocity sufficient to carry it into the air for enough time that it can be caught on the third cycle. Consequently, we see that both the tangential and vertical velocity increase steadily to a maximum at 0.28 seconds. The vertical velocity and acceleration show a transitional phase within this throw portion at 0.11

seconds, probably due to the upward motion being transferred from the forefinger and wrist to the more slowly accelerating arm. After the throw, the forefinger then slows down slightly to permit the ball to clear the hand, and while it is moving across the top of the arc.

The catch shows up as a sharp negative minimum in vertical acceleration at 0.38 seconds as the downward force of the moving ball is transferred to the hand and finger. Moreover, since the hand is also moving laterally at this point, and must transfer this motion to the ball, we see a strong peak in the tangential acceleration at 0.42 seconds. The hand then accelerates downward, reaching its maximum velocity at 0.48 seconds, when the ball is falling nearly vertically.

At this point we enter the setup phase where the ball is positioned for its launch. A sharp positive peak in vertical acceleration is caused by the arm muscles contracting to slow the ball prior to transferring it back across the body to the launch position. We see in Figure 12.1 that this transfer takes around 0.11 seconds, and is comparatively slow compared to the speed that we see in the postcatch phase between 0.42 and 0.52 seconds.

In summary, we see something of note happening at intervals as small as 0.06 seconds in a cycle of length 0.7 seconds. As in many biomechanical processes, such as speaking, writing, and playing the piano, the brain is able to control muscular systems on very short time scales.

12.4   The linear differential equation

As with handwriting, we model juggling via a second-order linear differential equation in velocity rather than in position. In other words, the velocity function $x'(t)$ is the basic function to be modeled. The model then remains unchanged if we change the origin of the measurements. Since our decision to make the average spatial coordinates equal to zero was rather arbitrary, and certainly not related to any intrinsic structure of the motor control system that we are aware of, having a model that is invariant under translations seems essential.

Unfortunately, the coordinate system that we are using is not likely to be "natural" from a motor control point of view, unlike the handwriting situation where lateral, vertical, and lifting movements have a good chance of being controlled independently. Indeed, why should we even assume that the brain uses rigid Cartesian coordinates at right angles that do not change with time? Certainly, there may be cross-talk between coordinates, so that what is happening for the lateral X-coordinate may depend on what is also going on for the vertical Z-coordinate, for example. We need, therefore, a more general form that will not change if we alter coordinate systems at a later point in our research when we have some better ideas about

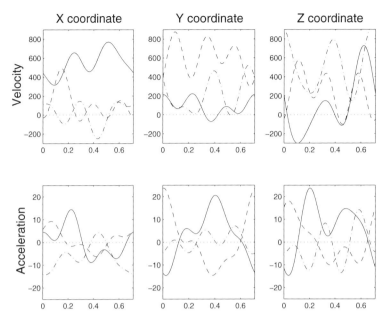

Figure 12.4. The top panels display the weight functions $\beta_{jk1}(t)$ on the three coordinate velocities for each coordinate. The bottom three panels show the acceleration weight functions $\beta_{jk2}(t)$. Within each panel, the X-coordinate weight function is the solid line, the Y-coordinate weight is the dashed line, and the Z-coordinate weight is the dashed-dotted line.

coordinates intrinsic to motor control, and that will allow for properties of one coordinate of velocity to be influential on another.

Consequently, we move to a *coupled* differential equation, while retaining linearity. This means that the change in each coordinate and its derivatives is considered to involve counterpart changes in each other coordinate. Here is the more general equation that we used:

$$x_{ij}'''(t) = \sum_{k=1}^{3} [\beta_{jk1}(t)x_{ik}'(t) + \beta_{jk2}(t)x_{ik}''(t)] + f_{ij}(t) \quad \text{for } j = 1, 2, 3. \quad (12.3)$$

Note that i indexes replications and both j and k index coordinates. For coordinate j, regression coefficient weight functions $\beta_{jj1}(t)$ and $\beta_{jj2}(t)$ correspond to those given in the model (12.1) above. But for this jth coordinate we also have the four cross-coordinate regression coefficient weight functions $\beta_{jk1}(t)$ and $\beta_{jk2}(t)$, $k \neq j$. There are, therefore, a grand total of 18 weight functions to be estimated. This might seem like a lot, but remember that we have 123 juggling cycles at our disposal.

Figure 12.4 shows the weight functions $\beta_{jk1}(t)$ and $\beta_{jk2}(t)$ that we estimated. The estimation method is outlined in Section 12.6 below. The resulting estimated forcing functions correspond to residuals in standard

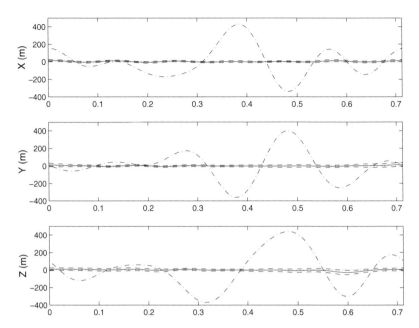

Figure 12.5. The panels display the mean forcing function $\bar{f}_j(t)$, 95% pointwise confidence limits for this function, and, for reference purposes, the mean jerk function $\bar{J}_j$ for each coordinate. The solid line close to zero is the mean forcing function, the dashed lines on either side are 95% pointwise confidence limits, and the dashed-dotted line is the mean third derivative, displayed to indicate the relative size of the forcing function.

statistical modeling, and Figure 12.5 gives one assessment of the fit of the model, showing that the mean forcing function is much closer to zero than the mean jerk function for each of the coordinates. Another measure of fit is obtained by noting that, for each coordinate and for all t, over 99% of the variability in the jerk function is explained by the model.

What features do the estimated weight functions display? These functions were estimated using a Fourier basis with seven basis functions, which permits precisely three cycles, and in most cases the variation at this scale is clear. Allowing more cycles produces almost no improvement in fit, but on the other hand the fit deteriorates if fewer basis functions are allowed. This suggests that there is genuine detail in the brain's control mechanism at cycle lengths of order a quarter of a second.

Were we right in allowing cross-talk between coordinates? Looking at the effect of velocity (the top three panels in Figure 12.4) we see that the jerk in each coordinate is clearly influenced by that coordinate's own velocity. However, the Z-velocity has a clear influence on the jerks in the X- and Y-coordinates, and all three velocities seem to affect the jerk in the vertical direction. The acceleration effects are less clearcut, but there is

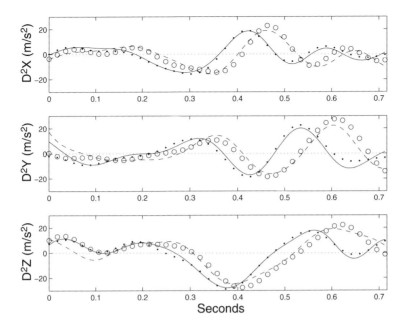

Figure 12.6. The fits to two sets of the coordinate acceleration functions based on the homogeneous linear differential equation. The fit and the actual data for the first record are plotted as a solid line and dots, respectively; and the results for a record from the middle of the juggling sequence as a dashed line and open circle, respectively.

no sense in which the effects of the different coordinates are disentangled. Confirmatory evidence of the need to allow influence between coordinates was provided by attempting to fit separate differential equation models to each coordinate; the quality of fit was much lower.

The fit of the equation to the data can be explored further by solving the homogeneous version of differential equation (12.3) for each coordinate, using the estimated weight functions β_{jk1} and β_{jk2}. There are six linearly independent solutions for the velocity functions, and every solution can be expressed as a linear combination of these. The solutions can each be thought of as a basis function, or mode of variation, in juggling cycle space, in rather the same way as the harmonics in principal components analysis. We may then approximate each of the 123 actual cycle curves or their derivatives by expanding them in terms of these functions. In approximating the curves themselves, we use the condition that the mean position is zero to recover the absolute position from the velocity. If a cycle is well modeled by the equation we would expect it to be well approximated by these basis functions.

Figure 12.6 shows how well the acceleration curves $x''_{ik}(t)$ are fit for the first cycle and for a cycle drawn from the middle of the sequence. The fits shown are fairly typical for all cycles. Similar quality of approximation is also achieved for both position and velocity. Thus, the equation does a fine job of capturing both the curve shape for an individual record and its first two derivatives. Moreover, the six basis functions seem to do a good job of following the variation in the shape of the observed functional data from replication to replication.

12.5   What have we seen?

We saw in Section 12.3, and especially in Figure 12.3, that there are three main phases in the juggling cycle: throwing, catching, and setting up the next throw. Each phase lasts around 0.24 seconds. The tangential acceleration curves seem to display some cyclical features with approximate cycle lengths multiples of 0.12 seconds. This quasiperiodic character of acceleration has been observed in a wide variety of situations in neurophysiology, for example by Ramsay (2000) in the study of handwriting. It leads us to suspect that the motor control system uses a basic clock cycle to synchronize the contractions of the large numbers of muscles involved in complex tasks.

Our main modeling tool was the linear differential equation discussed in Section 12.4. We used this type of model because we already saw how important the acceleration curves were in describing the juggling process, and we wanted an approach that provided a good model of velocity and acceleration as well as the observed position data. Also, linear differential equation systems are the backbone of models in mechanics and other branches of engineering and science, and they should prove useful for describing biomechanical systems such as this. All the Fourier cycles used in the fitting of the weight functions shown in Figure 12.4 have cycle lengths that are multiples of 0.12, but this would not have been the case if a richer Fourier basis were used. The good fit of the model with this property is certainly consonant with the motor control clock cycle hypothesis.

The data were fitted extremely well by a second-order linear homogeneous differential equation, without any forcing function or nonlinear effects. The six modes of variability corresponding to the solutions of this equation fit individual juggling cycles extremely well and also allowed for the variation from one juggling cycle to another. In a certain sense, there is no variation between cycles; they are all controlled by the same differential equation, suggesting that the process of learning to juggle is one of "programming" a suitable differential equation into the person's motor system.

It is beyond the scope of this chapter to attempt to discern what coordinate system the brain is using to plan movement. Preliminary investigations involving eigenvalue analyses of the matrices of coefficients β suggest that the coordinate system remains relatively stable during parts of the cycle, and then changes as different muscle groups come into play. This, and several other aspects of our model fitting, are fascinating topics for future research.

12.6   Notes and references

The juggling study was carried out in collaboration with Dr. Paul Gribble of the University of Western Ontario in the motor control laboratory of Prof. David Ostry at McGill University.

Chapter 14 of Ramsay and Silverman (1997) gives more detail of the underlying methodology of this chapter, but only for the case of a one-dimensional variable rather than a space curve. We fit the model (12.3) by an integrated least squares procedure, the natural extension of the method set out in their Section 14.2. The criterion of fit of the functions β is to minimize the integrated residual sum of squares

$$\text{IRSE} = \int \sum_{i,j} [f_{ij}(t)]^2 dt$$

$$= \int \sum_{i,j} \left\{ x_{ij}'''(t) - \sum_{k=1}^{3} [\beta_{jk1}(t)x_{ik}'(t) + \beta_{jk2}(t)x_{ik}''(t)] \right\}^2 dt \quad (12.4)$$

The fit is regularized by constraining each β to have an expression in terms of a fairly small set of basis functions. In the juggling context, a seven-term Fourier expansion was used because of the periodicity of the problem; an alternative would be a B-spline basis on a fairly coarse knot sequence. The number of basis functions controls the degree of regularization, and other regularization approaches are possible.

In the present context, there are 18 β functions to be estimated, and hence $7 \times 18 = 126$ basis coefficients altogether. Substituting the basis expansions into (12.4) gives an expression for IRSE as a quadratic form in these 126 coefficients. The matrix and vector defining this quadratic form are found by numerical integration, and standard numerical techniques then yield the estimated coefficients.

References

Bock, R. D. and Aitkin, M. (1981). Marginal maximum likelihood estimation of item parameters: Application of an EM algorithm. *Psychometrika*, **46**, 443–459.

Cleveland, W. S. (1979). Robust locally weighted regression and smoothing scatterplots. *Journal of the American Statistical Association*, **74**, 829–836.

Craven, P. and Wahba, G. (1979). Smoothing noisy data with spline functions. *Numerische Mathematik*, **31**, 377–390.

Dempster, A. P., Laird, N. M., and Rubin, D. B. (1977). Maximum likelihood from incomplete data via the EM Algorithm. *Journal of the Royal Statistical Society*, Series B, **39**, 1–38.

Dryden, I. L. and Mardia, K. V. (1998). *Statistical Shape Analysis*. Chichester: John Wiley & Sons.

Falkner, F. T. (Ed.) (1960) *Child Development: An International Method of Study*. Basel: Karger.

Gasser, T. and Kneip, A. (1995). Searching for structure in curve samples. *Journal of the Americal Statistical Association*, **90**, 1179–1188.

Gasser, T., Kneip, A., Ziegler, P., Largo, R., and Prader, A. (1990). A method for determining the dynamics and intensity of average growth. *Annals of Human Biology*, **17**, 459–474.

Glueck, S. and Glueck, E. (1950). *Unraveling Juvenile Delinquency.* New York: The Commonwealth Fund.

Green, P. J. and Silverman, B. W. (1994). *Nonparametric Regression and Generalized Linear Models: A Roughness Penalty Approach.* London: Chapman and Hall.

Harman, H. H. (1976). *Modern Factor Analysis.* Third edition revised. Chicago: University of Chicago Press.

Hastie, T. and Tibshirani, R. (1993). Varying-coefficient models. *Journal of the Royal Statistical Society,* Series B, **55**, 757–796.

Hastie, T., Buja, A., and Tibshirani, R. (1995). Penalized discriminant analysis. *Annals of Statistics,* **23**, 73–102.

Hermanussen, M., Thiel, C., von Büren, E., de los Angeles Rol. de Lama, M., Pérez Romero, A., Ariznaverreta Ruiz, C., Burmeister, J., and Tresguerres, J. A. F. (1998). Micro and macro perspectives in auxology: Findings and considerations upon the variability of short term and individual growth and the stability of population derived parameters. *Annals of Human Biology,* **25**, 359–395.

Johnson, R. A. and Wichern, D. W. (2002). *Applied Multivariate Statistical Analysis.* Fifth edition. New Jersey: Prentice Hall.

Kneip, A. and Gasser, T. (1992). Statistical tools to analyze data representing a sample of curves. *Annals of Statistics,* **20**, 1266–1305.

Kneip, A., Li, X., MacGibbon, B., and Ramsay, J. O. (2000). Curve registration by local regression. *Canadian Journal of Statistics,* **28**, 19–30.

Leth-Steenson, C., King Elbaz, Z., and Douglas, V. I. (2000). Mean response times, variability, and skew in the responding of ADHD children: A response time distributional approach. *Acta Psychologica,* **104**, 167–190.

Leurgans, S. E., Moyeed, R. A., and Silverman, B. W. (1993). Canonical correlation analysis when the data are curves. *Journal of the Royal Statistical Society,* Series B, **55**, 725–740.

Lord, F. M. (1980) *Application of Item Response Theory to Practical Testing Problems.* Hillsdale, N.J.: Erlbaum.

Lord, F. M. and Novick, M. R. (1968). *Statistical Theories of Mental Test Scores.* Reading, Mass.: Addison-Wesley.

Malfait, N., Ramsay, J. O., and Froda, S. (2001). The historical functional linear model. McGill University: Unpublished manuscript.

Mardia, K. V., Kent, J. T., and Bibby, J. M. (1979). *Multivariate Analysis.* New York: Academic Press.

Ramsay, J. O. (1995). A similarity-based smoothing approach to nondimensional item analysis. *Psychometrika*, **60**, 323–339.

Ramsay, J. O. (1996a). A geometrical approach to item response theory. *Behaviormetrika*, **23**, 3–17.

Ramsay, J. O. (1996b). Principal differential analysis: Data reduction by differential operators. *Journal of the Royal Statistical Society*, Series B, **58**, 495–508.

Ramsay, J. O. (1998). Estimating smooth monotone functions. *Journal of the Royal Statistical Society*, Series B, **60**, 365–375.

Ramsay, J. O. (2000). Functional components of variation in handwriting. *Journal of the American Statistical Association*, **95**, 9–15.

Ramsay, J. O. and Bock, R. D. (2002). Functional data analyses for human growth. McGill University: Unpublished manuscript.

Ramsay, J. O. and Dalzell, C. (1991). Some tools for functional data analysis (with discussion). *Journal of the Royal Statistical Society*, Series B, **53**, 539–572.

Ramsay, J. O. and Li, X. (1998). Curve registration. *Journal of the Royal Statistical Society*, Series B, **60**, 351–363.

Ramsay, J. O. and Silverman, B. W. (1997). *Functional Data Analysis.* New York: Springer-Verlag.

Ramsay, J. O., Bock, R. D., and Gasser, T. (1995). Comparison of height acceleration curves in the Fels, Zurich, and Berkeley growth data. *Annals of Human Biology*, **22**, 413–426.

Rice, J. A. and Silverman, B. W. (1991). Estimating the mean and covariance structure nonparametrically when the data are curves. *Journal of the Royal Statistical Society*, Series B, **53**, 233–244.

Roche, A. F. (1992). *Growth, Maturation and Body Composition: The Fels Longitudinal Study 1929–1991.* Cambridge: Cambridge University Press.

Rossi, N. (2001). *Nonparametric Estimation of Item Response Functions Using the EM Algorithm.* M.A. thesis, Department of Psychology, McGill University.

Rossi, N., Wang, X., and Ramsay, J. O. (2002). Nonparametric item response function estimates with the EM algorithm. McGill University: Unpublished manuscript.

Sampson, R. J. and Laub, J. H. (1993). *Crime in the Making: Pathways and Turning Points Through Life*. Cambridge, Mass.: Harvard University Press.

Shepstone, L. (1998). *Patterns of Osteoarthritic Bone Change*. Ph.D. thesis, University of Bristol.

Shepstone, L., Rogers, J., Kirwan, J., and Silverman, B. W. (1999). The shape of the distal femur: A palaeopathological comparison of eburnated and non-eburnated femora. *Annals of the Rheumatic Diseases*, **58**, 72–78.

Shepstone, L., Rogers, J., Kirwan, J., and Silverman, B. W. (2001). The shape of the intercondylar notch of the human femur: A comparison of osteoarthritic and non-osteoarthritic bones from a skeletal sample. *Annals of the Rheumatic Diseases*, **60**, 968–973.

Silverman, B. W. (1982). On the estimation of a probability density function by the maximum penalized likelihood method. *Annals of Statistics*, **10**, 795–810.

Silverman, B. W. (1985). Some aspects of the spline smoothing approach to non-parametric regression curve fitting (with discussion). *Journal of the Royal Statistical Society*, Series B, **47**, 1–52.

Silverman, B. W. (1995). Incorporating parametric effects into functional principal components analysis. *Journal of the Royal Statistical Society*, Series B, **57**, 673–689.

Silverman, B. W. (1996). Smoothed functional principal components analysis by choice of norm. *Annals of Statistics*, **24**, 1–24.

Simonoff, J. S. (1996). *Smoothing Methods in Statistics*. New York: Springer-Verlag.

Thalange, N. K., Foster, P. J., Gill, M. S., Price, D. A., and Clayton, P. E. (1996). Model of normal prepubertal growth. *Archives of Disease in Childhood*, **75**, 427–431.

Tuddenham, R. D. and Snyder, M. M. (1954). Physical growth of California boys and girls from birth to eighteen years. *University of California Publications in Child Development* **1**, 183–364.

Wang, X. (1993). *Combining the Generalized Linear Model and Spline Smoothing to Analyze Examination Data*. M.Sc. thesis, Department of Statistics, McGill University.

Whittaker, E. (1923). On a new method of graduation. *Proceedings of the Edinburgh Mathematical Society*, **41**, 63–75.

Index

2PL model, 135
3PL model, 136

ability space curve, 132–135
acceleration of stature, 86–89
ADHD, 7–8, 69–79
adult crime level
  as principal component, 28–31
agonist, 146
American College Testing Program,
  131
amplitude variation, 10, 91–96,
  101–114
analysis of variance (ANOVA), 74–76
antagonist, 146
arc length
  as nonlatent trait, 140–143
  parameterization by, 117–120
arthritis, 6, 10–11, 57, 62–63, 120–130
attention deficit hyperactive disorder,
  see ADHD
average shape, *see* mean shape

basis expansions
  definition, 33–35

fitting to observed data, 35–36, 60,
  106
for bivariate regression function,
  150
for log density, 80
for periodic trend, 107
for periodic weight function, 178
for relative acceleration, 98
for univariate regression function,
  151
principal components as, 125
Berkeley Growth Study, 84, 98
bimodality of reaction time
  distributions, 72
biomechanics, 57, 65, 128, 170
bone shapes, 6–7, 10–11, 57–66,
  115–130
B-splines, definition, 34–35

canonical correlation analysis, 129
charting variable, 134
Choleski decomposition, 38
climate data, *see* weather data
coarticulation, 145
condyle, 58
contemporary linear model, 149
coupled differential equations, 177

crime data, 3–4, 17–18
criminology, key issues, 4
cyclical spline interpolation, 60

density estimation, 80–81
Depression, the Great, 43, 48–49
depressor labii inferior muscle (DLI),
        146
desistance
    as principal component, 28
    definition, 17
differential equation model, 54,
        162–165, 176–180
differential item functioning (DIF),
        139
difficulty of a test item, 135
discrete values
    turning into functional data, 19–21
discriminability of a test item, 135
discriminant analysis, 123–130
dynamic linear model
    for classification, 166–169
    for handwriting, 162–165
    for juggling, 176–180
    general introduction, 158–160

eburnation, 57
economic data, see nondurable goods
        index
electromyography, see EMG
EM algorithm, 136
EMG, 146
evaluation point, 35

fair score, 139
false negative, 130
false positive, 130
feedforward model, 147
Fels Institute, 83
finite element method, 150
forcing function, 160, 162, 164, 178
F-test
    of functional linear models, 155
functional canonical correlation
        analysis, 129
functional data analysis
    definition, 15
functional discriminant analysis, see
        discriminant analysis

functional linear model, 148
functional linear regression, 148
functional mean, 21
functional observations
    independence assumptions, 3, 15
functional parameter of growth, 90
functional principal components
        analysis, see principal
        components analysis

gender differences
    in growth, 94
    in test performance, 138–140
goods index, see nondurable goods
        index
growth
    functional parameter of, 90
growth spurt, 84

handwriting, 9–10, 101, 104–105,
        157–170
harmonic motion, 159
harmonic process, 45
harmonics, see principal components
        analysis
high desistance/low adult score
        (HDLA), 30–31
historical linear model, 149
homogeneous differential equation,
        160

infrared emitting diode (IRED), 172
intercept function, 148, 160
intercondylar notch, 58
intrinsic metric, 141
irregular data, 36
item characteristic curves, 134
item response function, 134

jerk function, 162, 171
juvenile crime level
    as principal component, 28

kinetic energy, 45–46

landmark-free methods, 116–120
landmarks, 59–60, 115
latent trait, 134

least squares, penalized, *see* roughness penalty smoothing
leaving-one-out error rate (for classification), 130, 166
life course data, 17–19
linear discriminant analysis, *see* discriminant analysis
linear regression, functional, *see* functional linear regression
lip acceleration, 146–147
loading vector, 23
log densities, 74
log odds-ratio function, 135–138
logistic model, 135–136
long-term desistance
    as principal component, 28
longitudinal data, 17
LOWESS smoother, 156

mean shape, 61, 120
mean, functional, 21
midspurt, 89
monotone curve
    differential equation for, 89–91
    estimation by penalized likelihood, 98–99
Mont Royal, 103
motoneuron, 145
motor control, 157, 171–172
multimodality, 76–77

neural control of speech, 145
nondurable goods index, 4–6, 41–56
nonhomogeneous differential equation, 160
nonlatent trait, *see* arc length
nonparametric density estimation, *see* density estimation

odds ratio, 135
OPTOTRAK system, 172
osteoarthritis, *see* arthritis
outlines, *see* shapes

paleopathology, 57
patellar groove, definition, 58
PCA, *see* principal components analysis
penalized EM algorithm, 136

penalized maximum likelihood density estimation, 72, 80–81
    see also roughness penalty smoothing
periodic cubic spline, 60
phase variation, 10, 91–96, 101–114
phase-plane plot, 5, 44–47
physiological time, 92
polygonal basis, 34
potential energy, 45–46
prepubertal growth spurt, 87, 89, 94–96
principal component scores, 23
principal components analysis
    algorithm for functional, 37–38
    of densities, 76–79
    of growth curves, 95–96
    of log odds-ratio, 136–138
    of shape variation, 61–65, 120–123
    of warping function, 95–97
    regularized, 26
    scatter plots of components, 28–29
    unsmoothed, 23–25, 61
    varimax rotation, 63–65
    visualizing components, 25, 27
principal differential analysis, 13, 163
probability density estimation, *see* density estimation
Procrustes transformation, 61
pubertal growth spurt (PGS), 84

registration, 91–96, 101–114
regularization
    by restricting the basis, 181
    of discriminant analysis, 125–127
    see also roughness penalty smoothing
relative acceleration, 90
resubstitution error rate (in classification) 130
roughness penalty smoothing
    based on fourth derivative, 55
    for log density functions, 80
    for mean function, 21
    for monotone functions, 98–99
    for warping functions, 113–114
    in PCA context, 26
    in terms of basis functions, 36

saltation, 86
scores, *see* principal component scores
Second World War, 41, 42, 48, 50
shape variation
  principal components of, 61–65,
      120–123
shapes
  definition of mean, 61, 120
  parameterization of, 59–60, 117
simple harmonic motion, 45, 159
smoothed sample mean, 21–23
  algorithm for, 36–37
smoothing parameter choice
  cross-validation, 38–40
  informed subjective choice, 23, 26,
      55–56, 81, 91, 99, 113–114
space curve, 132
speech, 145
spline interpolation, 60
St. Lawrence River, 103
St. Peter's Church, Barton-upon-
      Humber, 57
stature
  acceleration of, 86–89
  measurement of, 83–84
stock market crash, 41
system time, 102

tangential acceleration, 104–105, 173
tangential velocity, 173
temperature patterns, 105–110
three-parameter logistic model, 136
time deformation function, 108–109
time series, functional, 6
time warping, *see* registration
triangular basis, 34, 150–151
two-parameter logistic model, 135

variance-stabilizing transformation,
      21
varimax rotation
  definition, 63–64
  vector form, 67
varying coefficient model, 156
Vietnam War, 48

warping, *see* registration
weather data, 105–110
Web site, 2

weight vector, 23

Springer Series in Statistics *(continued from p. ii)*

Küchler/Sørensen: Exponential Families of Stochastic Processes.
Le Cam: Asymptotic Methods in Statistical Decision Theory.
Le Cam/Yang: Asymptotics in Statistics: Some Basic Concepts, 2nd edition.
Liu: Monte Carlo Strategies in Scientific Computing.
Longford: Models for Uncertainty in Educational Testing.
Mielke, Jr./Berry: Permutation Methods: A Distance Function Approach.
Pan/Fang: Growth Curve Models and Statistical Diagnostics.
Parzen/Tanabe/Kitagawa: Selected Papers of Hirotugu Akaike.
Politis/Romano/Wolf: Subsampling.
Ramsay/Silverman: Applied Functional Data Analysis: Methods and Case Studies.
Ramsay/Silverman: Functional Data Analysis.
Rao/Toutenburg: Linear Models: Least Squares and Alternatives.
Reinsel: Elements of Multivariate Time Series Analysis, 2nd edition.
Rosenbaum: Observational Studies, 2nd edition.
Rosenblatt: Gaussian and Non-Gaussian Linear Time Series and Random Fields.
Särndal/Swensson/Wretman: Model Assisted Survey Sampling.
Schervish: Theory of Statistics.
Shao/Tu: The Jackknife and Bootstrap.
Simonoff: Smoothing Methods in Statistics.
Singpurwalla and Wilson: Statistical Methods in Software Engineering:
    Reliability and Risk.
Small: The Statistical Theory of Shape.
Sprott: Statistical Inference in Science.
Stein: Interpolation of Spatial Data: Some Theory for Kriging.
Taniguchi/Kakizawa: Asymptotic Theory of Statistical Inference for Time Series.
Tanner: Tools for Statistical Inference: Methods for the Exploration of Posterior
    Distributions and Likelihood Functions, 3rd edition.
van der Vaart/Wellner: Weak Convergence and Empirical Processes: With
    Applications to Statistics.
Verbeke/Molenberghs: Linear Mixed Models for Longitudinal Data.
Weerahandi: Exact Statistical Methods for Data Analysis.
West/Harrison: Bayesian Forecasting and Dynamic Models, 2nd edition.

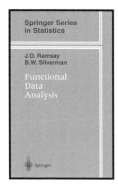
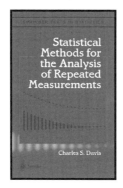
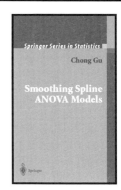
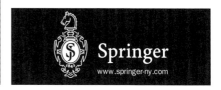